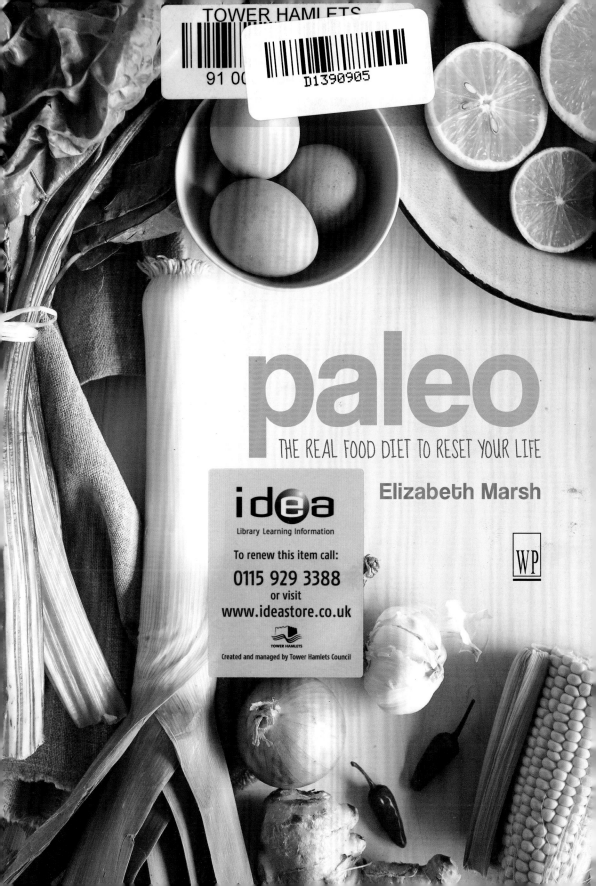

paleo

THE REAL FOOD DIET TO RESET YOUR LIFE

Elizabeth Marsh

WP

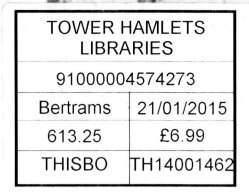

Published by:
Wilkinson Publishing Pty Ltd
ACN 006 042 173
Level 4, 2 Collins St Melbourne,
Victoria, Australia 3000
Ph: +61 3 9654 5446
www.wilkinsonpublishing.com.au

International distribution by Pineapple Media Limited
(www.pineapple-media.com)   ISSN 2203-0832

National Library of Australia Cataloguing-in-Publication entry

Author: Marsh, Elizabeth Jane, author.

Title: Paleo : the real food diet to reset your life / Elizabeth Marsh.

ISBN: 9781922178558 (paperback)

Subjects: Diet therapy--Popular works.
Nutrition--Popular works.
Food habits--Popular works.
Self-care, Health--Popular works.

Dewey Number: 613.2

Layout Design: Tango Media Pty Ltd
Cover Design: Tango Media Pty Ltd

Photos by agreement with Rachel Jane Cam.

PRIMAL
JUNCTION

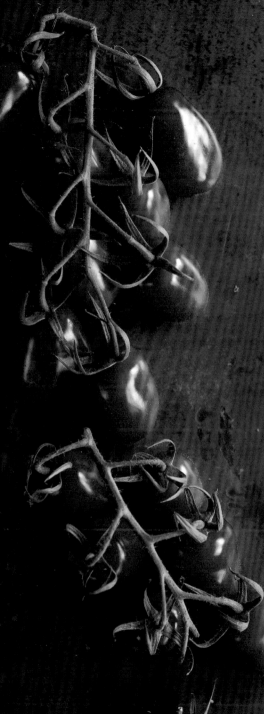

Contents

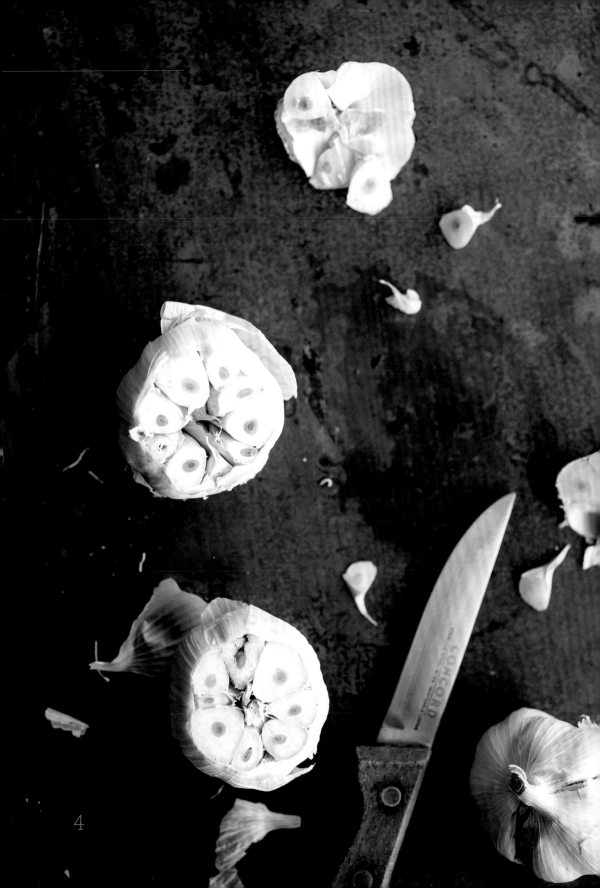

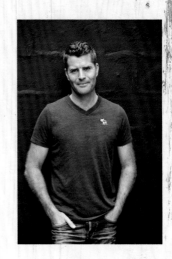

FOREWORD

I think we can all agree that food is medicine or food is poison depending on what we choose to put on the end of our fork, spoon or chopsticks —or if you are living the caveman way, what you eat with your fingers.

Never before in history has there been so much talk about what we should or shouldn't eat. Unfortunately the messages are so confusing and every day another claim is made, often distorted by the media to suit their demographics or to keep their advertisers happy. Thankfully the Paleo diet is a practical voice that has risen above the noise in the last decade or two, thanks to the amazing work of passionate and brilliant minds such as Boyd Eaton, Loren Cordain and Nora Gedgaudas, to name a few, who have shone a bright light on what can only be called a common sense and evolutionary science based approach to our optimal eating and health plan.

I myself have been following a Paleo lifestyle for the last 3 years; my own transformation has been nothing short of astounding and I am still constantly learning what is best for my body.

The fact that we now have the global culinary pantry open to us with the abundance of spices, herbs, seafood, meats, fruits and veggies like never before means that we now have the ability to create an astonishing array of healthy meals for ourselves which is literally endless. I have never viewed Paleo as restrictive but instead, utterly indulgent with the choices I now have to play with. I am positive that once you embrace this way of life—as this is what Paleo is all about, a new lifestyle—that you will never turn back, as the energy you will have will be unlike anything before.

Lizzy outlines the dos and don'ts and whys and hows very simply in the following pages and I am sure you will love cooking the delicious recipes that are part of the Primal Junction cookbook... Bon appétite and keep cooking and eating with love and laughter.

Pete Evans
www.thepaleoway.com

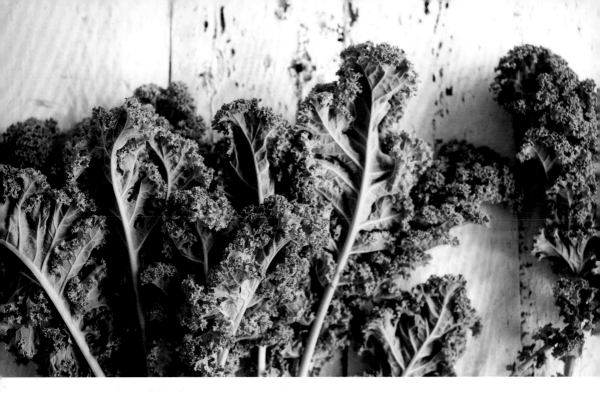

INTRODUCTION

Paleo is an opportunity for me to combine my ideas around nutrition, health and lifestyle with the goal to educate and inspire you to live a life you love. After studying in the fields of medicine and exercise science, I became frustrated with the symptom-based and pharmaceutical approach to illness and disease and wanted to learn more about achieving optimal health and athletic performance from the angle of illness prevention. I want to share my knowledge with others so that we can all access our full potential as human beings and live a life of purpose, vitality and fun.

Before my own drastic lifestyle change, I thought I was really healthy. I was following the nutritional guidelines and eating large servings of whole grains, fruits and low-fat foods. I was heavily involved with regular endurance exercise while training for a half Ironman triathlon and was training hard in an attempt to reduce body

fat and still be able to eat the foods that I was supposed to. I became frustrated with fluctuations in body weight and was finding that little injuries were constantly popping up, as well as muscle tightness, fatigue and an overall exhaustion. My times weren't improving and I found it increasingly difficult to keep my eyes open at university lectures. The constant energy crashes and recurring sicknesses meant that I could never be consistent with my training. Although I still thought I was 'healthy,' I knew that something had to change, and fast.

My journey started with an abrupt 30-day self-experiment to completely remove potentially inflammatory and reactive foods from my diet and re-set my digestive system, allowing for repair and regeneration. This was also an opportunity for me to start to learn how to listen to my body and question how it felt in response to a range of food types. I realised that I had eaten many of these foods for so long that I could no longer recognise how they were impacting my health. I reduced my endurance-training load and avoided all processed foods. I began filling my plate with large salads, clean protein and piles of vegetables.

After this experience, I have never looked back. I felt more alive and in tune with my body than ever. Over the 30-day period, I lost 4-5 kilograms (9-11 pounds) of body fat, slept more soundly, had boundless energy throughout the day, clearer skin and an overall enthusiasm and zest for life. I also had a LOT of questions.

Over the last three years, I have explored and researched the Paleo approach and have established a nutrition and lifestyle consulting business, Primal Junction, to share my love of real food with others. I hope that this book will provide you with the tips, tricks, recipes and inspiration to live a life that you love fuelled on real-food. Most of all, I hope that I can encourage you to question the accepted nutritional and health guidelines and take control of your own life by asking questions, experimenting and standing for your health from this moment forward!

WHAT IS PALEO?

The Paleo diet refers to the diet consumed by our ancestors starting some 2.5 million years ago and ending with the start of the agricultural revolution about 10,000 years ago. During this Palaeolithic era, humans lived in small tribes and hunted and gathered their food. Although there were variations depending on location, environment and climate, research shows that these diverse primitive diets consisted mostly of small and large game, fish, vegetables, tubers, fruits, and nuts. Lacking were the grains and legumes, not to mention refined sugars and oils, as seen in modern diets.

With the invention of agriculture, communities were able to start producing larger volumes of food, leading to the industrial revolution and the exploration of refined oils and production of sugar. Along with the influx of these highly refined foods came the onslaught of 'diseases of the Modern Age' such as cardiovascular disease, diabetes, cancer, high blood pressure and obesity. Today, these diseases are affluent in all Western communities and the situation doesn't appear to be improving.

In the Palaeolithic era, food was a necessity and research demonstrates that we did not always have enough of it. Today, what to cook for dinner is one of the most troubling and confusing questions, with an infinite number of answers provided by professionals, online sources, books and nutritional bodies. With unlimited access to processed and refined foods it can be difficult for many to question the modern nutritional guidelines and marketing of industrial food products and get back to basic, real food from small, sustainable community sources.

Contrary to popular belief that early humans lived brutal and dangerous lives with short life expectancies, our early relatives were in fact lean, fit and strong with similar aerobic fitness, body composition and blood pressure values to modern-day trained athletes. Life expectancy values that are commonly used to debate this way of life are in fact skewed by infant mortality rates and early death caused by trauma and injury instead of illness and disease. Even in modern times, there are societies and tribes that are still nourishing themselves by hunting and gathering, with no access to processed food or modern medicine. For example, members of the Hunza tribe from the mountain peaks in the Himalayas frequently live to the age of 130 or greater, and at these ages, still live vibrant, active and high quality lives.

By reconnecting with real food and being conscious about illness prevention, we can re-define what it is to be a human in the modern world. With access to both nourishing and healthful foods, and conventional medical research you can be a lean, physically fit and powerful human being with a zest for life that will extend into old age.

In summary, the Paleo diet is about eating foods that we are genetically designed to eat and that have made up our natural diets for over 2 million years, while avoiding processed and refined foods that have been introduced much more recently. In general, this way of eating avoids processed foods, refined sugar, commercial dairy products, grains and refined oils. Instead, we pile our plates high with high quality and diverse meats, poultry and seafood, lots of vegetables, nuts, seeds, fruits, eggs and high quality saturated fats like coconut oil.

THE MODERN CAVEMAN

Many readers associate the Paleo diet with the carnivorous, harsh and un-hygienic lives of our cave-dwelling ancestors. At first mention of the world 'Paleo', long-haired cavemen equipped with spears and loincloths immediately come to mind. However, the Paleo lifestyle is not about trying to re-enact human life as it was 2.5 million years ago. It's about exploring a real-food and holistic approach to life without the processed and refined foods of the modern world that can be linked to marked increases in disease. It is also about supporting your local communities and knowing the individuals who provide and supply your food. It's about voting with your dollar to promote ethical and sustainable business practice.

Living a Paleo or Primal life is all-encom-passing. It's holistic. It's about eating what we're genetically able to process and moving your body in ways that we are designed to move. For our ancestors, movement involved actions like squatting, throwing, hanging, swinging, climbing, pulling, pushing, jumping and lifting. To reach optimal health in the modern world, we need to re-define what it means to be human, reconnect with our natural movement patterns and fuel our bodies with natural foods.

THIS IS NOT A WEIGHT-LOSS PROGRAM OR SHORT-TERM 'FIX'

The Paleo lifestyle is a way of reducing the intake of foods that may be negatively impacting our body and adding more healthful foods into our day. After a lifetime of processed dairy products, chemicals, sugars, refined foods and poor quality ingredients, many people are no longer sensitive to how foods are making them feel. A poor quality diet can be reflected in a vast array of symptoms that we have accepted as 'normal life.' These might include fatigue, mid-afternoon tiredness, digestive problems, bloating, bad skin, chronic pain, anger and frustration, and a loss of vitality or lack of excitement for life.

The Paleo diet takes into account those foods that may be causing an underlying immune response (when our body thinks we are sick and fighting an intruder) and focuses on adding foods that will contribute to muscle growth, fat loss, reduced inflammation, acid/alkaline balance, nutrient density and satiety. The most exciting part is that the Paleo diet does not involve counting calories, food restric-tion or diet foods and supplements. It is based on eating foods that are recognised by the body with a low level of immune response and inflammation for the majority of the population. By normalising our blood sugar and incorporating a diverse array of nutrient dense foods, you will bounce out of bed in the morning and feel energised and excited about what you can achieve each and every day. This book will not provide you with a set meal plan or strict rules. Achieving a long-term, sustainable and healthy relationship with food is about discovering what works for your body, lifestyle and budget.

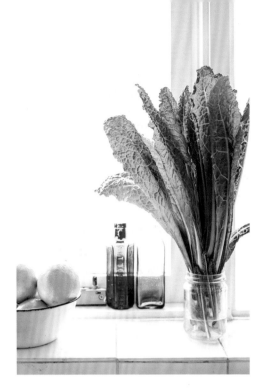

THE SCIENCE BEHIND THE FOODS WE EAT

One of the easiest ways to look at the principles behind eating Paleo and the way that different foods interact within our body is to separate food groups into those that are making us healthier and those that *may* be making us less healthy.

The word *may* is important. As individuals, we all interact with foods differently. For some of us, ingesting dairy products is accompanied by bloating, digestive problems and pain. For others, there are no apparent symptoms. For each of us, there is a scaled level of intolerance to those foods that we were not genetically designed to consume and the body interacts, presenting numerous symptoms that vary from person to person. The important thing to remember is that these symptoms can show up in a range of ways for different people, from skin conditions to afternoon energy slumps, so sometimes the impact of our diet will slip by unnoticed. It is also important to realise that no 'diet' or eating plan will have the same impact on every person. Eating Paleo is a template. The information presented is designed to inspire you to *question* the accepted nutritional and exercise

guidelines that constantly bombard us from the health industry. The best way to know if something works for you is to try it for yourself. Be consistent, experiment, listen to your body and provide it with the opportunity to 'reset'.

This section will address some of the underlying physiological changes that occur throughout our day to day activities, and also how different foods will make us feel depending on how they are broken down and utilised by the body. By understanding some of the physiological processes, it is often easier to embrace changes to your lifestyle and make the first steps towards cleaning out your pantry!

INFLAMMATION

Inflammation is one of the most important areas to address when wanting to lose body-fat, improve performance or boost your health. Inflammation is not only directly related to the foods that we eat, but also to our hormones, stress levels, type of exercise and lifestyle. Although we generally think of it as a negative reaction to an injury or illness, inflammation is a natural response by the body as a way to protect itself from infection, injuries and intruders. For example, acute inflammation is the redness, swelling and heat that occurs when you cut your finger and is a critical stage in the repair process. Inflammation can become a little less helpful when things go wrong and the body starts to illicit an immune response much more often than it needs to (or chronically), resulting in issues like acne, fatigue, allergies, poor gut health, ulcers, rheumatoid arthritis, asthma, inflammatory bowel disease and more.

Systemic inflammation occurs when chronic inflammation moves beyond the tissues and into the lining of blood vessels and organs. This type of inflammation infiltrates the whole body and places it in an activated immune response state that circulates the blood stream. Long-term systemic inflammation has been shown to wreak havoc on our health and immunity, increasing the risk of developing many modern diseases such as insulin resistance, diabetes, high blood pressure, cardiovascular disease, obesity, neurological conditions and digestive ailments like irritable bowel syndrome (IBS).

As our lives become busier and busier, lifestyle factors that may increase inflammation are on the rise. For many of us, inflammatory foods, busy jobs, high stress, chronic endurance exercise, coffee addictions and processed diets all contribute to the "inflammatory bucket" and it is becoming increasingly important to focus on reducing our level of inflammation to combat this survival mode and allow us to live a big life without the increased risk of disease and burnout.

There are many lifestyle factors that result in an inflammatory response, but not as many that can reverse this state. One of the main influencers on the level of inflammation (and one of the only things we have total control over!) is our diet. Foods can either contribute to our inflammatory response by eliciting an immune response in the body, or help to reduce inflammation by providing us with maximal nutrition and minimal reaction. One of the main benefits of the Paleo

Inflammation – the silent illness

One of the main issues with systemic inflammation is that it's a silent condition – we may not know that we have it, and the indicators can present themselves as a range of different signs and symptoms that vary from person to person. So how do you know if you're inflamed?

Here's a brief checklist that should give you a little indication.

✔ I eat grains
✔ I eat processed dairy products
✔ I am overweight
✔ I carry extra body fat around my abdomen (stomach)
✔ I eat processed foods
✔ I drink alcohol
✔ I eat refined sugar
✔ I'm constantly exercising
✔ I'm often stressed

This doesn't include the long list of ailments, signs and symptoms that are indicators too. Inflammation can be responsible for acne, illnesses, osteoporosis, joint pain, fatigue, depression, asthma, migraines, chronic pain and much, much more.

diet is that the majority of these inflammatory foods are avoided, giving our immune system a chance to rest, re-set and repair.

IMMUNE RESPONSE

Our level of inflammation is somewhat controlled by our immune system. Designed to fight 'intruders' and protect the body from bacteria, parasites, viruses and fungi, this complex system will react and attack visitors that are identified as 'non-self.' The easiest entry point for most of these bad guys is straight into our digestive system via the mouth. If we are constantly eating foods that our body doesn't recognise, like refined sugars, chemicals and inflammatory foods like gluten-containing grains and legumes, an immune response is generated to fight and protect. For many people, the body is in a constant state of fighting and reactivity, leading to compromised immunity. When a serious virus or stressful event presents itself, this baseline inflammation and activation means that the body is over worked and unable to maintain optimal health.

ACID/ALKALINE BALANCE

Food is so much more that just 'healthy' and 'unhealthy.' Above and beyond the immune and inflammatory responses to foods, it is important to also understand that the acid/base content of foods can affect your health. The human body's top priority is to maintain balance (or homeostasis). When we eat foods that are acid –forming (the average Western diet is slightly acidic), the kidneys are involved with registering this change and the body will buffer to bring the pH levels back to normal. Over time, this acid load on the kidneys can cause problems such as

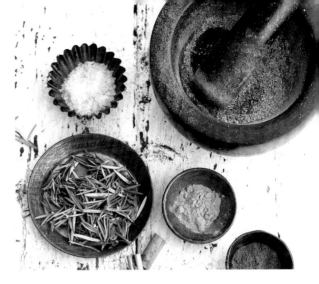

bone and muscle loss with aging, and calcium and other mineral deficiencies.

We need both acidic and alkaline foods to achieve balance. When most people remove the 'filler' foods like grains, bread and dairy products from their diet and focus on eating high quality proteins and fats, they sometimes make the mistake of not re-filling their plate with alkaline foods like piles of vegetables and some fruit.

FOODS TO AVOID

SUGAR
Refined and added sugar is omitted from the Paleo diet for a number of reasons. Not only have we developed processed and refined sugars that far exceed the sweetness found in nature, we have surrounded ourselves with this highly addictive and nutrient-void product.

In the Palaeolithic era, sugar was an extremely rare find. Our ancestors loved honey and were prepared to fight bees to get their hands on it. Other than the occasional beehive, refined carbohydrates were non-existent and even the sugars found in fruits were much less intense. Consider the taste of a wild crab-apple compared to a sweet and juicy Pink Lady!

When we did find sugar, our metabolic processes were designed to make the most of it. The high fructose (a specific form of sugar) content in honey meant that we could eat as much as possible without registering the 'full' centres in our brain. In this era, this was part of survival. The rarity of energy dense foods meant that we needed to store as much as possible for later use. Have you ever wondered why you can eat a whole bag of candy or drink a litre of orange juice without getting full? This 'save it for later' mechanism might explain why.

Fructose metabolism bypasses the brain and heads straight to the liver where it can be stored for later use, or is released into the blood stream as free fatty acids. Problems arise when we "find a beehive" all day long, constantly producing free fatty-acids and burning the constant supply of energy in our bloodstream rather than the fat that we have stored. Excess energy in this form is stored as body fat. Therefore, rather than blaming dietary saturated fats for our obesity epidemic, it makes more sense to make the connection between a drastic increase in refined sugar intake and the storage of excess energy as body fat.

As well as the reliance on sugar instead of fat for fuel, continual 'sugar hits' throughout the day mean that we need to secrete more of the hormone insulin to regulate blood sugar levels. Over time, excess production of insulin can

What about fruit?

Although modern fruits are a *lot* sweeter than those gathered by our ancestors, they are still a real-food in their whole form. Fruit is a living, natural plant. Although containing varied amounts of different types of sugars, fruit also contains fibre, water, vitamins, minerals and phyto-nutrients.

Depending on your body composition goals, excess fruit can also impact us in the same way as regular sugar-feeding throughout the day so just be aware that an apple for afternoon tea may fuel your addiction to the sweet stuff rather than help you break it. A great guideline is to always stick to fruits in their whole form and look for those that contain lower levels of sugar, particularly if you are insulin resistant or wanting to lose body fat. Eating some fats or protein with your fruit will also help to slow the insulin response of your snack or meal. For example, you could have a small handful of nuts or some slices of chicken breast with your afternoon fruit snack.

The table below shows a few examples of the higher and lower total sugar options (not necessarily ranked in order).

LOWER SUGAR FRUITS	HIGHER SUGAR FRUITS
Lemon and lime	All dried fruit
Avocado	Grape
Strawberry	Banana
Papaya	Mango
Grapefruit	Apple
Blueberry	Pineapple
Fresh fig	Pear

Source: Cordain, L, Fruits and Sugars, Sugar content of Fruits, http://thepaleodiet.com/fruits-and-sugars/

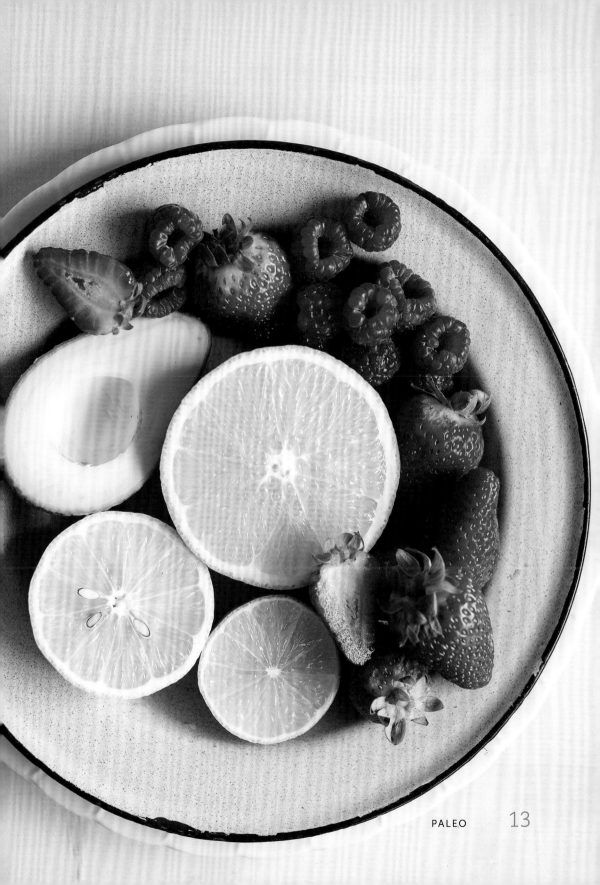

lead to insulin resistance, and in more severe cases, type 2 diabetes. By reducing our reliance on refined and potent sweeteners, we can control blood sugar with less insulin release and reduce the risk of developing these types of metabolic conditions.

For most of us, cutting sugar out of our diet isn't an easy task. The over-stimulation of our taste buds and pleasure centres means that it is harder and harder to satisfy cravings and almost impossible to appreciate the sweetness of foods like strawberries, carrots or vine-ripened tomatoes. The reward-response from sugar also means that it's highly addictive. When you stop your intake of sugar abruptly, your body suffers withdrawals and this can manifest as head-aches, fatigue, crankiness, frustration and poor performance.

After the initial period of suffering, normally around 5-7 days, our taste buds regenerate and the taste of food actually *changes*. You will start to taste the sweetness in fruits and vegetables and your body will not be on the lookout for sugary foods as a mid-afternoon pick-up. Soon, you'll feel fuller for longer as you'll be starting to rely on fats for fuel rather than regular sugar spikes. This also means that your blood sugar will stabilise, you'll have less excess carbohydrate to store as body fat and you'll bounce out of bed in the morning, ready to tackle the day.

SWEETENERS – REAL AND ARTIFICIAL

As more research surfaces and confirms the numerous health conditions and illnesses associ-ated with a high intake of refined sugars, an increasing number of sugar alternative products have become available on the market. Whether a sweet product is marketed as natural, raw, unrefined or calorie-free, sugar is sugar.

Both natural and artificial sweeteners will pro-vide a pleasure-response and fuel our reliance on

sweet foods and sugar-fixes without adding any nutritive value to our day. Artificial sweeteners are just that – artificial. They offer no nutritional value and are designed to make us believe that a food is sweet when it's not. The chemical processing of sweeteners like Nutra-Sweet, Equal, Splenda and stevia places them on the no-go list. In general, it's best to remove the majority of sugar (natural or artificial) from the diet and focus on sourcing carbohydrates from whole fruits and vegetables. When you consider the diet of our ancestors, sugar was not something consumed daily, or even weekly!

DON'T BE FOOLED

Sugar is added to many foods on the industrial food chain. Be sure to check the ingredients list of all foods and aim to buy those that don't need an explanation! Sugar is often disguised under many different terms, so we've distinguished some of the best options for you. If you are making the occasional sweet treat, choose these when you can and avoid other 'natural' and all artificial sweeteners as much as possible. Not sure how to use these sweeteners? Check the back of the recipe section for some cleaner sweet treat ideas.

- Dates (whole)
- Fruit (whole)
- Fruit juice
- Raw honey
- Maple syrup
- Molasses

DAIRY PRODUCTS

Most of the time, dairy products fall into the 'avoid' category on the Paleo diet. However there is a huge difference between the dairy products available on your supermarket shelves and those in their natural form. In the Palaeolithic era, dairy

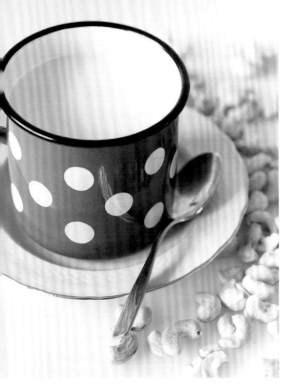

WHAT ABOUT CALCIUM?

It is a common belief that dairy products are the only source of calcium in our diet. This is just simply not true. Calcium is important for many cell processes, including muscle contraction when we exercise, and is present in high amounts in green leafy vegetables, seafood, nuts, fruits and vegetables.

The most important consideration, however, is the balance between calcium *excretion* and calcium *absorption*. This is intricately related to the acid-alkaline balance that was discussed earlier. Calcium and other important bone minerals are required to assist with the buffering process when we eat a diet high in acid-forming foods like cheeses, grains, dairy, meat and eggs. Instead of eating more foods high in calcium, we can decrease the amount of calcium that we excrete by consuming more alkaline foods. A Paleo diet high in alkaline vegetables and fruits neutralises the dietary acid caused by meat and seafood and reduces the risk of bone loss and osteoporosis. This balance is particularly important for athletes with a higher utilisation of minerals like potassium and calcium. Load up on fresh fruits and vegetables to promote strong bones, injury prevention and healthy muscle contraction.

REFINED OILS

The Paleo diet incorporates the use of healthy, naturally occurring and minimally processed fats and oils. There are a few important features of oils and fats to consider – their stability, smoke point and how they've been made.

Industrial oils like peanut, 'vegetable', sunflower, corn, canola and rice bran oil have been through a comprehensive refining process to convert seeds and grains into a cheap and highly reactive product. These oils are high in polyunsaturated fatty acids (PUFA)

products were not included in the diet beyond the mother's milk provided to an infant for fast growth and immunity.

When dairy products are prepared for supermarket shelves, the pasteurisation and homogenisation processes can destroy the nutritious and helpful bacteria, leaving an acid-forming and inflammatory food with not a whole lot of nutritional value. Many individuals are sensitive or even allergic to dairy – often diagnosed as lactose or casein protein intolerance. Even worse, low-fat dairy products are often full of sweeteners and artificial flavourings.

Some followers of the Paleo diet may decide to keep some forms of dairy in their day. This may be because they have a low reactivity or intolerance to products like full-fat, organic yoghurt, grass-fed butter or raw (unpasteurised and unhomogenised) milk. Of all the dairy products, these contain the highest amount of nutrition, healthy fats and helpful bacteria.

and omega-6 fatty acids – fats that have been shown to promote systemic inflammation and are highly unstable when heated due to a low smoke point.

Contrary to the nutritional guidelines over the last 30-40 years, high-quality saturated fats are in fact the best choice for storing, heating and eating to promote health, satiety and flavour. The connection between saturated fats and heart disease has been shown to be flawed, with research now uncovering many important factors such as fat quality, smoke points and other lifestyle factors like sugar and processed and refined food intake when considering heart disease risk.

Saturated fats, like coconut oil and animal fats are a stable and unreactive source of fatty acids. These fats can withstand higher cooking temperatures and will last a lot longer in your pantry. They do not become rancid easily, and are therefore the best choice for cooking and baking.

The table below summarises the fats and oils to choose for both hot and cold uses, as well as the industrial products to dispose of when you clean out your pantry. Make sure all fat sources are organic, pasture-raised, grass-fed, extra-virgin, cold-pressed and sustainable (check the food quality section for more info).

SATURATED – FOR HEATING	UNSATURATED – FOR COLD USE	POOR QUALITY – DISPOSE
Coconut oil	Extra-virgin olive oil	Margarine
Palm oil	Sesame oil	Canola oil
Butter	Macadamia nut oil	Corn oil
Ghee	Walnut oil	Grape seed oil
Meat	Avocado oil	Rice bran oil
Seafood	Flaxseed oil	Rapeseed oil
Animal fats (bacon, tallow, duck fat)	Nuts	Sunflower oil
Full fat dairy	Seeds	Safflower oil
Eggs	Nut and seed butters	Soybean oil

High-quality saturated fats are the best choice for storing, heating and eating to promote health, satiety and flavour.

GRAINS AND LEGUMES

Removing grains is one of the biggest changes when people transition to a Paleo diet. This means no more breads, pasta, rice, cereals or corn (yes, corn is a grain!). This food group became a staple part of the human diet after the agricultural revolution, just 10,000 or so years ago, and is now recommended as one of our primary sources of carbohydrate. The main reason that grains and legumes are mostly avoided in a Paleo diet is not only because of the inflammatory response that they elicit, but also the low nutritional value contained within them. Grains offer no additional nutrition to fruits and vegetables, only providing higher inflammation, acidity and reactivity in most of the population. Legumes fall within the same category – for many individuals, it is extremely difficult to digest and break them down (which is why some people notice gas and bloating when they are consumed). For others, this reaction is not as noticeable, and particularly for those following a vegetarian diet, legumes can provide an alternative protein source.

What about fibre? Refined grains, whole grains and legumes are often advertised for their high fibre content, but it is just as easy and much less inflammatory to access this fibre from whole fruits and vegetables. For example, half of a sweet potato or one cup of green beans contains as much fibre as 1 cup of oats.

GLUTEN

Gluten is a protein composite found in several types of grains including wheat, rye, spelt and barley. Gluten is named after its glue-like texture and is a sticky protein that gives bread and pasta its elastic properties. The main problem with gluten is the reactivity that it can cause in the body. For individuals that are sensitive to gluten, particularly those that have been diagnosed celiac, gluten is treated in the body like a foreign invader. The immune system will turn on an 'attack' as a protective mechanism, which can lead to digestive discomfort, nutrient malabsorption, anaemia, fatigue and an increased risk of developing diseases like cancer, autoimmune diseases, anaemia, bowel disease, neurological diseases and more. In fact, a review paper in *The New England Journal of Medicine* listed 55 "diseases" that can be caused by eating gluten. There is no benefit to eating this inflammatory protein, and most people will find that they feel better without it in their diet. Often it is difficult to tell whether you react to gluten, as symptoms can be silent or unrecognisable because we are so used to feeling tired and bloated and have accepted this as 'normal' life.

SOY PRODUCTS

The Paleo diet excludes all soy products, both refined and fermented. Soybeans are legumes in their natural, raw state and are in fact poisonous and must be cooked. Similar to other legumes and grains, soybeans are high in phytates that reduce the bioavailability of nutrients.

The main reason to question and remove most soy products completely is related to the way in which they can interfere with estrogen receptors in the body and alter the natural control of this important hormone. Unfortunately soy products and their industrial by-products are present in a large amount of packaged foods and livestock feed. Soy most commonly appears in soybean oil, which is a highly reactive and refined oil high in non-favourable Omega-6 fatty acids that can have a negative impact on health when we over-consume them.

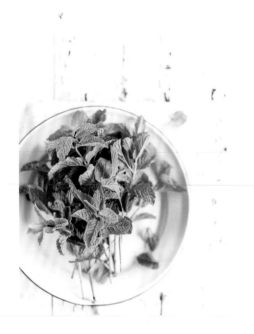

FOODS TO EAT AND WHY

Now to the exciting part! The best thing about the Paleo diet is all the delicious, nutritious and colourful foods that will fill your plate and provide you with the nutrients and energy to bounce out of bed in the morning and live a life that you love.

An important thing to remember when changing your eating habits and consuming a lot less "filler" foods like bread, pasta, rice and cereal, is to make sure that you're eating *enough*. One of the most common errors is to cut out these large food groups without replacing the energy provided by these foods with other sources. For example, if your breakfast normally consists of two pieces of toast with two eggs and a slice of bacon, you may be disappointed and hungry when you remove the bread and don't add anything in its place. In this situation, there are a number of ways to bulk up your plate with nutrient dense foods that will keep you full for longer. Instead of inflammatory and energy dense

toast, pile up your plate with some sweet potato fritters (page 52), vegetables, half a grapefruit, fresh berries or cauliflower 'rice' (page 84).

FATS

Fats are an extremely important part of a healthy diet. Fats contribute to our hormone health, skin health and immunity. The primary sources of fats in the Paleo diet come from animal fats, clarified butter, ghee, fish oils and seafood, avocados, olives, eggs, coconut products and some nuts and seeds.

By consuming healthy fats with each meal, we can teach our bodies to burn fats more efficiently as a fuel when we're walking, cleaning, cooking and at work. This means that we can burn more body fat at low intensities. For some endurance athletes, a higher fat diet will allow them to utilise this energy dense fuel source and preserve their carbohydrate stores for later in a race or when it's needed most.

FAT QUALITY

When we focus on real, whole foods, it is also important to address food quality and to know

> Although contrary to the "saturated fat causes heart disease" debate, a meta-analysis compiled by the *Journal of Clinical Nutrition* looked at 21 studies that followed more than 300,000 participants for up to 24 years, tracking saturated fat intake and incidence of heart attack and stroke. They found no significant evidence to conclude that dietary saturated fat intake is linked to an increased risk of coronary heart disease, stroke or cardiovascular disease.
>
> Source: Hartwig, D and M, *It Starts with Food*,
> Victory Belt Publishing, 2012.

where our fuel sources are coming from. This includes purchasing foods without health claims and nutrition labels, and voting with our dollar to support local butchers, grocers and farmer's markets. Ideally, we'd be switching over to local, organic, seasonal and well-raised sources, but sometimes this can involve an increase in food costs. There are certain considerations that may have a bigger impact on your health than others, so I'll recommend how to make this transition a little easier and more affordable.

Fats are particularly important when considering food quality, as many of the toxins, pesticides, hormones and chemicals that are used to produce higher volumes of food more cheaply are fat-soluble, meaning that they are 'held' and stored within an animal's fatty tissue. This is also the case for dairy products like butter and ghee – organic and grass-fed sources will contain fewer toxins than commercially available supermarket products. Just like they're held in an animal's fatty tissue, these toxins can be stored and build up in our own tissues too. If you don't have access to grass-fed, organic sources of meat, we recommend that you trim the fat before cooking and eating. With cleaner sources of meat, there's no problem with eating the fatty trim!

Nuts and seeds are another source of fatty acids on the Paleo diet. As with all foods however, we need to make sure that we're eating these nuts in their most natural form. As nuts are high in unsaturated fats, their delicate oils can be damaged easily. It's best to go for raw, organic nuts that are from local sources if possible. Often nuts that are imported can be fumigated or treated. To increase the bioavailability of nuts and to make them more digestible, soaking before use is ideal to remove some of the nutritional inhibitors and toxins.

PROTEIN

Protein is an important macronutrient for recovery, repair, satiety and many chemical processes that take place in the body. Protein is involved with enzyme formation, and is therefore a critical component for processes like digestion, metabolism and DNA repair.

On the Paleo diet, dietary protein sources come from meat (both farmed animals and wild game), seafood and eggs.

PROTEIN QUALITY

As with fats, the *quality* of our protein sources is critical to reaching optimal health. With the goal to prepare and consume foods that are closest to their natural form as possible, it becomes important to address how our protein sources are fed and raised. For example, if a cow that is genetically designed to graze on grass is raised on a grain-based diet, this will impact the quality of the meat, health of the animal and inevitably the health of those who are consuming its meat. Not only does the meat taste better and support a sustainable and more environmentally friendly industry, meat from grass-fed animals has a superior nutrient profile, with more Omega-3 fatty acids, less impact from stress hormones and more micronutrients and vitamins, like vitamin A precursor beta-carotene and vitamin E.

The same goes for eggs. Chickens that are raised on an un-natural diet high in grains, hormones and supplements will produce a lower quality egg than those that are 'pasture raised' and allowed to roam and graze on worms and insects. Many conventional eggs come from chickens that never go outside and are raised in cages to promote mass-production of poor quality eggs.

The best way to ensure that you are supporting ethical, sustainable and healthy farming practices is to ask! Ask your local butcher about their sources of meat. Find out what chickens are fed, visit farms and request change. If we can all ask more questions and stand for the health of our animals, food and community, we can vote with our dollar to change the way that animals are farmed and our food is treated.

CARBOHYDRATES

Although many believe that the Paleo diet is a low or no-carbohydrate diet, it's possible for most individuals to reach adequate carbo- hydrate needs through the large amounts of both simple and complex carbohydrates found in real-food. Many current diets or eating plans have created a fear or negative attitude towards carbohydrates and sugars, when in fact they are a critical ingredient for a healthy human diet and were a sought after energy source for our hunter-gatherer ancestors. The problems arise when we consume refined and artificial sweeteners in excess. Healthy carbohydrates, contrary to most nutritional guidelines, are those that are as close to their natural form as possible, easily digestible and full of bio-available nutrients. Carbohydrates are extremely important to provide energy for exercise, important physiological functions and for fuelling important organs like the brain. For all these processes to take place however, the micronutrients, vitamins and minerals involved must also be present in the body. For this reason, when we eat carbohydrates in the form of refined sugar, like in a soft drink, this takes an inflammatory toll on the body rather than providing it with the nutrients and energy required to train hard or live a big life.

Our carbohydrate needs depend on the amount of energy we utilise throughout the day. For example, a person that is sedentary for most of the day will require a lot less fuel than an athlete who is training twice per day. When we

eat carbohydrate (no matter what form it's in), our body will use this energy first, preventing us from tapping into the energy dense fat stores that many of us would like to make use of! When we eat too much carbohydrate, excess is easily and efficiently stored as body fat. When we eat too little, particularly for active people, we can feel sluggish, tired, and irritable and may experience plateaus in performance.

There are a range of carbohydrates that all have a different effect on the body and the resulting blood sugar response. On the Paleo diet, our main carbohydrate sources come from dense high-carb vegetables and fruits. The list below includes some of the real-food vegetables that are highest in carbohydrate. For athletes, these foods are great to reach for as part of a post-workout meal to refuel muscle glycogen (stored energy).

As mentioned previously, fruits in their whole form are also a great carbohydrate source on the Paleo diet. To ensure that we

FOOD	CARBOHYDRATES PER 100G
Yam	27g
White potato	22g
Sweet potato	21g
Parsnips	17g
Beetroot	10g
Onion	10g
Carrot	10g
Butternut squash	10g
Spaghetti squash	6g
Pumpkin	5g

Source: Sanfilippo, D, *Practical Paleo*, Victory Belt Publishing, 2012

get all the fibre and nutrients that come with them, blending them or eating them whole is a preference over juicing. Mix up your fruit and vegetables as much as possible to ensure that you have access to a wide range of nutrients, vitamins and minerals.

CARBOHYDRATE QUALITY

When you purchase your weekly fruits and vegetables, a good question to consider is "how close is my food to its natural state?" This includes genetic modification and chemical sprays added to fruit and vegetables. Buy organic produce as much as possible from a local, sustainable and seasonal source. If this is not achievable, local produce is preferred over conventionally grown and genetically modified products. Check your local environmental governing body for information about the most heavily sprayed "dirty dozen" and least contaminated foods. In general, wash all fruit and vegetables really well and peel any conventionally grown produce that you can. Better yet, grow your own food. Lettuce, herbs and green leafy vegetables are a great place to start and will generally grow easily and in small spaces.

YOUR OWN PALEO DIET

There is no one diet or eating plan that will suit every individual. Whether you're training for a marathon, working towards better digestive health or fighting an illness or disease, the Paleo diet can be adapted to suit your goals and your lifestyle.

When working with individual clients to address their nutrition, inflammation and body composition goals, I recommend that they experience a 30-day 're-set.' This is a 30-day protocol or challenge that is similar to an elimination diet. The re-set allows your digestive system

to rest and repair while reducing the intake of inflammatory foods allows the immune system to take a break from its reactive state. It encourages us to consume the cleanest foods possible, and experience what life is like without a constant influx of refined foods.

After the 30-day re-set, it is interesting to start to add back in some of the foods that you may want to experiment with, like some forms of dairy, grains or legumes. This protocol allows you to become aware of how these foods make you feel and most people never go back to allergens like wheat, gluten and sugar after discovering how these impact their energy levels, digestion and overall health. Experiment with your own body, meal plans and lifestyle. Find out what makes you bounce out of the bed in the morning and what foods slow you down and make you sluggish.

TOOLS OF THE TRADE

All recipes in this book are easy, fast and delicious ways to fill your plate with nourishing, whole foods and without refined, processed and potentially harmful ingredients. Cooking for the Paleo diet is fun, sometimes challenging and always rewarding. There are endless Paleo recipe sources available both online and in books, and magazines. The more you cook, the more you will learn to substitute certain ingredients and work with a creative flair to turn your old favourites into clean, primal alternatives.

The following gadgets are some of the *extra* tools that will assist you in creating all the recipes provided in the book, and are helpful additions to any Paleo kitchen. No devices on this list are necessary, but are just nice to have!

A powerful blender: A high quality blender is a great tool for liquid recipes like smoothies, soups, nut butters, milk alternatives and drinks.

A food processor: Food processors with a couple of different bowl sizes will be your go-to for dips and marinades, ice-cream alternatives, sweet treats, mashes and puréed vegetables.

An immersion or hand-held stick blender: These are fantastic small devices that you can take with you! They are also the easier option for in-the-pot pureeing and soup-making. This gadget will make Paleo mayonnaise in a matter of seconds.

Slow cooker (crock pot): A slow cooker is particularly valuable in cooler months, when you want to come home to a nourishing, warm and tender meal. Slow cookers can be large enough to make big stews, curries and soups for dinner, with plenty of leftovers!

Pressure cooker: This appliance is fantastic if you want to cook tender meals in less than half the time. By cooking at a high pressure, this large pot will cook sweet potato in less than 10 minutes and a delicious fall-off-the-bone pot roast in about 40 minutes. These are great for those that get home from work and want to prepare a slow cooked meal in less than an hour.

Vegetable spiraliser: Vegetable spiralisers are a big hit in our kitchen. They are amazing tools that can turn vegetables into spiralled noodles, a great alternative for pastas. If you'd rather something smaller, a hand-held julienne device will make vegetable 'noodles' out of vegetables like carrots and zucchini too.

Microplane: These fine graters are ideal for fresh ginger and lemon zest, often called for in primal recipes and real-food cooking.

Ice-block moulds: These are handy little tools when you have kids at home, or if you like to have a frozen treat in the freezer over summer. Look for BPA-free plastic moulds and it's best if they have little drinking straws to help with melting pops!

PANTRY GUIDE

We recommend that clients kick off their re-set or dietary change with a big clean out of the pantry. If you're taking the step toward a Paleo lifestyle and better health, make the commitment and remove all processed or tempting foods while you make the initial adjustment. Check the nutrition panel of every product and if there's added sugar or nasty chemicals that you don't recognise – throw it away. If it's been in your pantry for longer than 6 months, it probably needs to go.

This will open up so much space for new, clean ingredients and staples. As we want to focus on real-food, you might find that your pantry is a little more spacious than before!

The initial swap from high-preservative and industrial foods to cleaner, organic and higher quality options can sometimes come with a hefty bill. Remember, you don't need all the things on this list at once. If you transition slowly and purchase one or two items with each shop you won't be spending big; without high ticket purchases like cereal, muesli bars and confectionery, you should be able to work these products into your budget. Remember, this is an investment in your health – your reduced medical bills will make up for it in the end!

This is just a brief summary of things you can incorporate into your diet but the options are endless and creativity in the kitchen is your best friend!

PANTRY SHOPPING LIST

OILS AND FATS	IDEAL OPTIONS
Extra virgin olive oil for cold uses	Organic, extra-virgin and cold-pressed
Macadamia nut oil for medium cooking temperatures	
Coconut oil for high heat grilling, frying and baking	
Grass-fed butter for medium cooking and baking	Organic, from grass-fed cows
Ghee or clarified butter	Organic
Nuts and nut butters (peanuts excluded as they are a legume, not a nut!)	Raw, organic and without other ingredients
Coconut cream and coconut milk	Organic with no strange ingredients. Look for BPA free cans and 100% kernel extract.

SAUCES + CONDIMENTS	IDEAL OPTIONS
Coconut aminos: similar to soy-sauce but gluten and wheat free	Organic
Tahini: ground sesame seed paste	Can be hulled or un-hulled
Mustard	Avoid added sugar, corn starch or oils
Pasta sauce	Avoid added sugar, flavourings and preservatives
Passata (tomato puree)	Avoid additives and sugar
Tomato paste	Organic and without preservatives
Apple cider vinegar	Organic or biodynamic
Hot sauce	Avoid added sugar
Pesto	Avoid poor quality oils or make your own

If you're taking the step towards a Paleo lifestyle and better health, make the commitment and remove all processed and tempting foods.

SPICES + SEASONINGS

SPICES + SEASONINGS	IDEAL OPTIONS
Moroccan or Cajun seasoning	Sugar and preservative free
Dukka/harissa	
Curry powder	
Ground cinnamon	Look for Ceylon cinnamon
Cumin	Organic and preservative free
Garam masala	
Turmeric	
Paprika	
Nutmeg	
Chilli	Fresh or chilli flakes
Ginger	Grated, fresh ginger is best
Salt: so many varieties! Smoked, seasoned etc	Choose pink Himalayan salt or ground sea salt

ADDED EXTRAS

ADDED EXTRAS	IDEAL OPTIONS
Coconut flakes	Organic, with no preservatives or additives
Desiccated coconut	
Goji berries: delicious chewy texture	
Cacao powder: high in magnesium	Raw
Cacao nibs: chocolate hit	Raw
Apple puree	Look out for added sugar and preservatives
Probiotics	Sauerkraut, fermented vegetables and kombucha
Stock cubes	Make your own or look for organic without preservatives.
Frozen berries and fruits	Organic

EAT WHOLE FOODS	ELIMINATE PROCESSED FOODS
VEGETABLES	**GRAINS**
The Paleo diet promotes pretty much all types of whole, organic, fresh vegetables. Discover a wide range of local and seasonal veggies to get access to a diverse range of vitamins and micronutrients.	Remove both whole and refined grains like cereals, breads, pasta, rice, wheat, barley, quinoa, millet, buckwheat and corn.
FRUITS	**PROCESSED FOODS**
Aim for lots of different varieties of fruit. Choose lower sugar fruits for a smaller blood sugar response.	Avoid all packaged and processed foods like muesli bars, pastries, protein bars, potato chips, candy, and chocolate bars. Look for hidden preservatives and chemicals.
PROTEINS (MEAT, SEAFOOD, EGGS)	**DAIRY PRODUCTS**
Choose meats from sustainable, grass-fed and organic sources when possible. Choose from a diverse range of meats including wild game, organ meats, and seafood. Look for organic eggs from pasture raised chickens.	Eliminate all processed dairy products including milk, yoghurt, cottage cheese, ice-cream and cheeses. Raw, unprocessed dairy is an option for some individuals.
NUTS AND SEEDS	**SWEETENERS**
As you start the Paleo diet, nuts can be a great snack option. However, they are easy to over-consume and can slow fat-loss results if this is your goal. Improve the nutrient absorption of your nuts and seeds by soaking them first.	Choose only natural, raw sweeteners in small amounts. This may include raw honey, maple syrup, dates and fruit. Avoid *all* processed and refined sugars including artificial sweeteners. Look for hidden sweeteners in most packaged goods!
FATS AND OILS	**REFINED OILS**
The quality of fats is very important when aiming to reduce the levels of toxins in the diet. Hormones, chemicals and toxins can all be stored in poor quality fats. For cooking, choose saturated fats like coconut oil, animal fats and ghee. For cold or low temperatures, choose nut oils and cold pressed olive oil.	Dispose of refined oils like margarine, sunflower oil, canola (rapeseed) oil, vegetable oil, rice bran oil and any old oils that have been exposed to light and/or high heats. Buy oils in small, dark bottles and keep them in a cool, dark cupboard or in the refrigerator.

Recipes

DRINKS
AND
SMOOTHIES

Beetroot and berry shake
Skin food green smoothie
Banana cacao bliss
Chai-spiced nut milk
Sugar-free iced tea
Coconut iced coffee
Fancy ice cubes
Anti-inflammatory ginger tonic
Hide the greens smoothie

Beetroot and berry shake

—— **SERVES 2** ——

Raw beetroot adds a shocking pink colour to any smoothie or shake. It has a wide range of health benefits, and has been particularly recommended for athletes wanting to improve their oxygen utilisation. Beetroot juice has been shown to decrease blood pressure within an hour of drinking! Its high nitrate levels have also been studied as a method of reducing the oxygen requirement of exercise and improving performance. In this recipe, we used homemade cashew milk but any milk substitute would work well too.

1 small beetroot, peeled

1 cup (250ml) cashew-nut milk

½ frozen banana

¾ cup (100g) frozen raspberries

1. Add all ingredients to the blender and pulse on high until smooth.

2. Top with a handful of frozen berries.

Make nut milk (page 34) with a variety of nut types. Make sure that you learn how to activate the nuts first to get the most nutritional value.

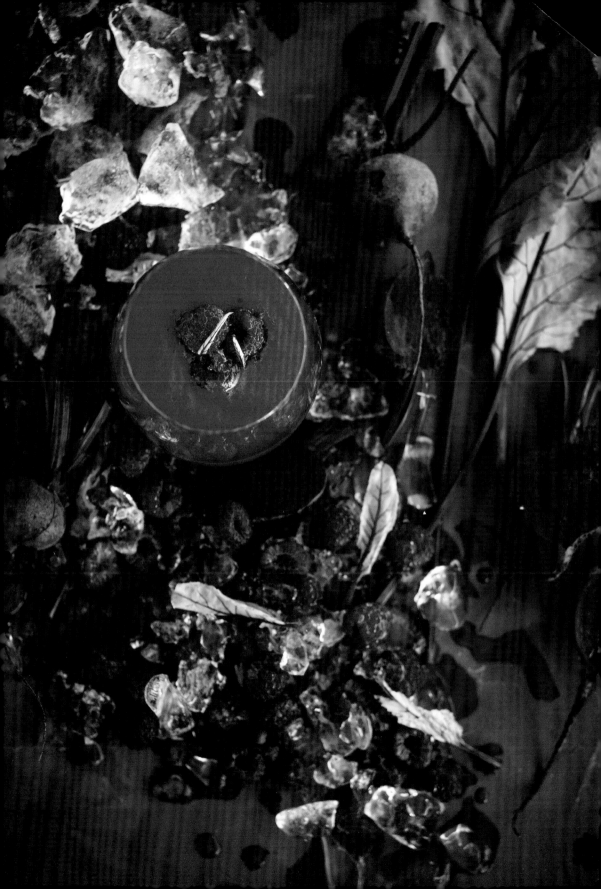

Skin food green smoothie

To me, true beauty is about health, happiness and a passion for life. One of the first places we notice this type of exuberant and energising beauty is in healthy, glowing skin.

This green smoothie is a creamy, delicious 'skin food'. With avocado, peppermint and coconut oil on the ingredients list, this smoothie is jam packed full of fatty acids, antioxidants and vitamins that will promote a healthy glow on the inside and out.

5 large kale (Tuscan cabbage) leaves, de-stemmed

½ avocado

1 lime, peeled

1 green apple, peeled and cored

½ cup (10g) fresh peppermint leaves (or mint)

1 tbsp coconut oil

3 ½ cups (875ml) filtered water

1. Wash all ingredients well.

2. Add all ingredients to your blender and blend on high for 90 seconds, or until smooth and creamy.

3. Serve with ice cubes and slices of fresh lime.

Banana cacao bliss

This recipe is a clean and creamy substitute for chocolate milk. If you have kids in the house this is an after-school treat that will give them a healthy dose of essential fatty acids, magnesium and carbohydrates to keep them satiated and fuelled up until dinner.

4 cups (1 litre) nut milk (page 34)

1 large frozen banana, without peel

3 tbsp raw cacao powder

½ tsp allspice

½ tsp pink Himalayan salt

½ tsp vanilla (or a couple drops of essence)

1. Add all ingredients to a blender or food processor.

2. Pulse until well mixed, thick and creamy.

3. Store in an airtight jug in the refrigerator and shake well before serving.

TIP: If you're currently adding protein powders to your diet, this is a great base to provide fats and carbohydrates for refuelling post-exercise.

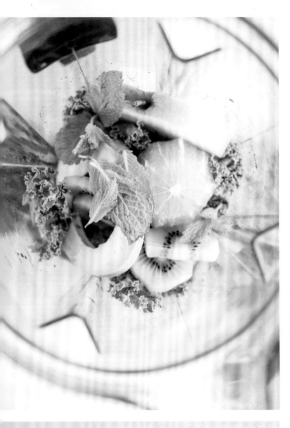

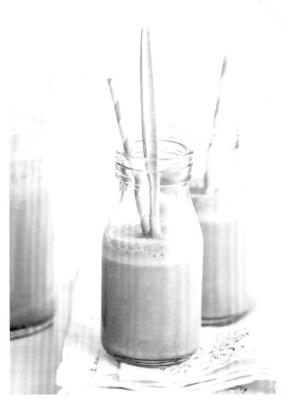

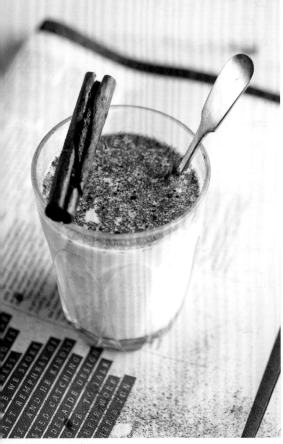

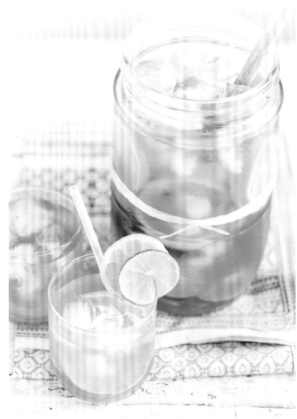

Chai-spiced nut milk

Milk is often one of the hardest products for people to remove from their diet. The pasteurisation of standard milk can destroy the beneficial bacteria, nutrients and enzymes found in raw milk. This process is a way of increasing the shelf life of a product that can be sold commercially. After exploring nut milks, I have found these are an even tastier start to the day and are a great source of protein and (depending on the nuts you use) magnesium, calcium and essential fatty acids.

This version of almond milk is infused with a natural chai tea mix, leaving a hint of warmth and sweetness that tastes delicious with the clean mean muesli (page 49). If you're looking for plain flavoured milk, omit the chai tea and soak the nuts by themselves.

1 cup (170g) raw nuts (cashews, macadamias or almonds work best)

2 tbsp loose leaf, sugar-free chai tea mix (or two tea bags)

4 cups (1 litre) filtered water plus extra for soaking

½ tsp vanilla bean (or vanilla extract)

Nut milk bag or cheese-cloth

1. Place the nuts and chai tea in a bowl and cover with filtered water. Cover the bowl and leave to soak overnight. With softer nuts like cashews and macadamias, you can get away with soaking them for just a few hours.

2. Drain the nuts and rinse well before adding to the blender with 4 cups of filtered water. You can adjust the amount of water to create a creamier or thinner milk.

3. Add a pinch of vanilla bean or dash of vanilla extract.

4. Blend on high for 90 seconds.

5. Place your nut milk bag or cheesecloth into a large bowl or jar and pour the milk into it. Squeeze it through to filter out the pulp. Creamier nuts like macadamias will have less pulp than others. Save the pulp from almonds to use as almond meal or in your next batch of bliss balls.

6. Store in the refrigerator in a glass, airtight container. Nut milks will last about 3-4 days.

WHY DO WE SOAK NUTS?

Raw nuts naturally contain phytic acid, which stores important nutrients by preventing them from sprouting. This is why raw nuts won't start growing in your pantry!

According to researchers, when consumed by humans, phytic acid reduces the body's ability to absorb many of these nutrients and the benefits contained in nuts are therefore less bio-available to us. Raw nuts also contain enzyme inhibitors that make the body work overtime to produce enzymes for digestion. This can place our digestive organs under strain and contribute to inflammation.

When we soak nuts, in a process called 'activation', germination is kick-started and both the phytic acid and enzyme inhibitors are broken down. In some ways this brings the nuts to life and makes the nutrients absorbable to the body. As we soak nuts for longer periods of time, the level of bio-available nutrients increases. To promote digestion and contribute to a nutrient rich diet, it is recommended that all raw nuts are soaked and then dried in a low oven, or dehydrated, before they are consumed.

Sugar-free iced tea

—— **MAKES 1 LITRE/4 CUPS** ——

Iced-tea is a refreshing alternative to soft drinks and juices that normally contain a high amount of sugar. You can use any tea; just check the ingredients list to make sure there are no hidden sweeteners or preservatives. You can freeze any leftover tea in an ice-cube tray or ice-block moulds for later.

1 cup (250ml) water

3 organic tea bags

1 lemon, sliced

20g (2 tbsp) fresh ginger, peeled and sliced

Ice cubes

Cold filtered water

1. Boil 1 cup of water.

2. Brew the tea bags for 2-3 minutes to make a concentrated tea.

3. Add the tea to a large jug with the lemon slices, ginger and two large handfuls of ice.

4. Top with cold water and fill with as much ice as possible.

Coconut iced coffee

2 shots black espresso coffee, cooled

¼ tsp vanilla extract

½ cup (125ml) cold water (or to taste)

3 tbsp coconut cream

1. Fill a large glass or jar with ice.

2. Add the coffee shots and vanilla. Stir to combine.

3. Add the cold water to desired strength.

4. Top with coconut cream before serving.

Fancy ice cubes

This is an efficient way to prevent wastage of bunches of fresh herbs or leftover lemons and limes. Get creative and use anything you like to spice up or sweeten your next soda water or iced tea.

Fancy ingredients
Filtered water

1. Chop, wash and prepare the fancy add-ins. Place some in each ice cube mould and top with water.

2. Freeze overnight or until solid.

Here are some fancy suggestions for ice cubes: chilli flakes, lemon and lime juice, mint leaves, lemon thyme, lavender petals, orange slices, ginger and berries.

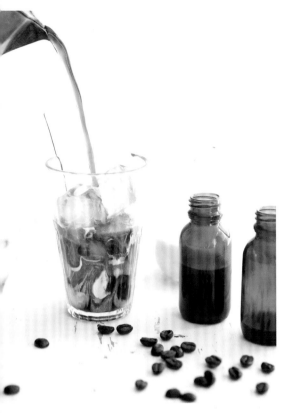

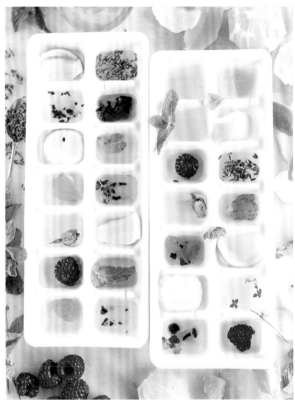

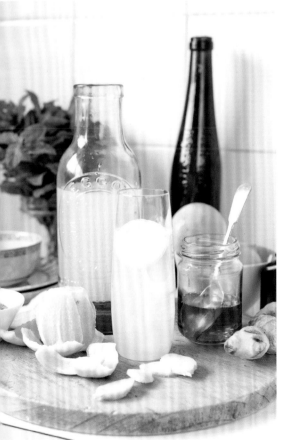

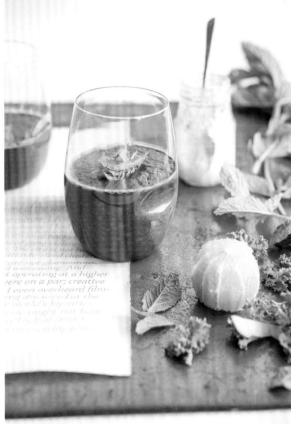

Anti-inflammatory ginger tonic

—— SERVES 3-4 ——

Start your day with a dose of this refreshing tonic full of anti-inflammatory gingerols and alkalising fresh lemon. If you're used to waking up and having coffee on an empty stomach, try some ginger tonic first to reduce acidity and kick-start digestion.

1 lemon, peeled

35g (3 tbsp) chunk of ginger, peeled (adjust depending on the strength you like)

4 cups (1 litre) filtered water

1 tbsp raw honey** (optional)

1. Add the lemon, ginger and water to your blender.

2. Blend on high until smooth (about 90 seconds).

3. If you want a pulp-free drink, pour the mixture through a nut milk bag* into your jug.

*If you don't have a nut milk bag, you can easily use a piece of muslin cloth or don't strain if you don't mind some ginger pulp.

**Honey has great antibacterial and anti-inflammatory properties so add a dash if you want to gently sweeten your tonic or if you're fighting a sore throat or cold.

INGREDIENT SPOTLIGHT

Ginger root is known to contain an abundance of potent anti-inflammatory substances called gingerols. For this reason, ginger is often used as a natural approach to the treatment of arthritis, joint pain and tendinitis and may in fact have a better therapeutic profile and fewer side effects than non-steroidal anti-inflammatory drugs. When we stress our system during endurance exercise, ginger may help to reduce systemic inflammation and inflammation linked to surrounding recurring injuries. Instead of reaching for a processed pharmaceutical option – why not try some of what nature has to offer?

Hide the greens smoothie

—— SERVES 2 ——

This smoothie is a great way to sneak some extra leafy greens into your day without even knowing it! Kale, like other members of the Brassica family, contains health promoting phytochemicals sulforaphane and indole-3-carbinol that appear to protect against a range of cancers such as prostate and breast cancers.

½ cup (85g) natural macadamia nuts

2½ cups (625ml) filtered water

1 cup (130g) frozen raspberries (or another frozen berry)

1 frozen banana

5-6 large kale (Tuscan cabbage) leaves

½ small beetroot, peeled

1. Soak macadamia nuts and water in a blender for 15 – 30 minutes to help soften the nuts.

2. Add the rest of the ingredients and blend on high for 90 seconds or until smooth.

3. Add water as required to reach your desired consistency. Garnish with mint leaves or frozen berries.

If you don't have access to kale, swap your leafy greens for something like spinach or silverbeet (Swiss chard)

BREAKFASTS

Rhubarb and apple crumble pots
Bacon and onion 'egg-ins'
Cashew cream
Chai-spiced poached pears
Holy-moly banana pancakes
Clean mean muesli
Chorizo and chilli frittata
Sweet potato fritters
Spicy steam-fried eggs on cauliflower rice

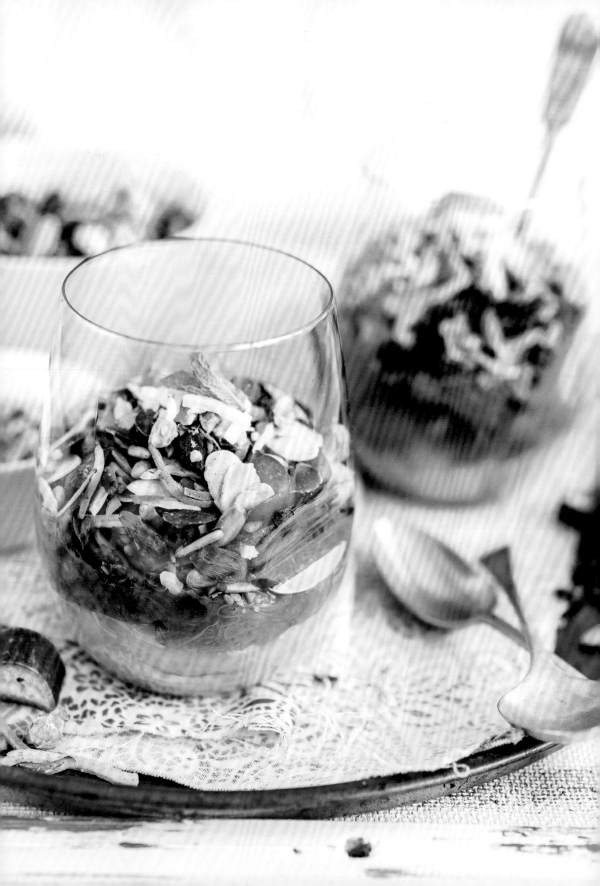

Rhubarb and apple crumble pots

—— SERVES 4 ——

On a Paleo diet, we remove a lot of the 'filler' breakfast foods like toast, cereal and yoghurt. In their place, we often reach for eggs as a staple protein. When we're in a rush or feeling like a lighter breakfast these crumble pots are a great alternative.

FOR THE FRUIT BASE

4 stems fresh rhubarb, leaves removed

400g canned pie apples* (check the ingredients to make sure it's 100% apple)

*If you don't have access to canned apples, make your own stewed apples by slow cooking chopped apple pieces until they soften.

FOR THE CRUMBLE

2 tbsp pepitas (pumpkin seeds)

2 tbsp sunflower seeds

2 tbsp sesame seeds

⅓ cup (40g) raw slivered almonds

⅓ cup (30g) shredded coconut

½ tsp Himalayan pink salt

½ tsp cinnamon

1 tsp chia seeds

¼ cup (25g) goji berries, roughly chopped

raw pistachio nuts, chopped

1. Wash and chop the rhubarb into small chunks. Add to a pot with about 3cm/1 inch of water. Bring to the boil then reduce to a low simmer until the rhubarb chunks start to soften and fall apart (about 15 minutes).

2. Allow the rhubarb to cool while making the crumble topping.

3. Into a dry pan over low heat, add the pepitas and sunflower seeds. Stir constantly as they lightly toast for about 2 minutes.

4. Add the sesame seeds, almonds, coconut, salt and cinnamon. Stir constantly as all ingredients are lightly toasted for another 2 minutes. Avoid high temperatures as this will cause the nut and seed oils to react and turn rancid.

5. Remove the nuts and seeds from the pan and place in a bowl to cool.

6. Once cooled, stir through the chia seeds and chopped goji berries.

7. In the bottom of a bowl or glass, place a layer of apple (about 3cm/1 inch thick).

8. Add a layer of stewed rhubarb of a similar thickness.

9. Top with a layer of crunchy crumble and a sprinkle of chopped pistachios.

TIP: Pre-make the fruit base and store in recycled jars in the fridge. On your way out the door or when you get to work, top with the crunchy crumble and enjoy.

Bacon and onion 'egg-ins'

12 slices of high quality streaky bacon

12 large eggs

4 spring onions (scallions), finely chopped

Smoked paprika

Chives, to serve

1. Preheat a conventional oven to 175°C / 350°F.

2. Cut baking paper into 12 7cm x 7cm (2.76 inches x 2.76 inches) squares and line a muffin tray with them.

3. Line the sides each muffin cup with a slice of bacon to create a ring. The bacon ring will hold the paper in place. Bake in the oven for 10 minutes or until crisp.

4. Meanwhile, crack eggs in a large jug, add the onion and mix well.

5. Remove the tray from the oven and pour the egg mixture evenly into the 12 bacon baskets. Don't worry if it goes outside of the bacon ring just aim to evenly fill the muffin holes.

6. Dust each egg-in with some paprika.

7. Bake at 175°C / 350°F for 25 minutes or until the tops are starting to brown and the egg is cooked through.

8. Sprinkle with chives to garnish.

Store the egg-ins for up to four days in an airtight container in the refrigerator. They are a perfect grab-and-go breakfast or daily snack.

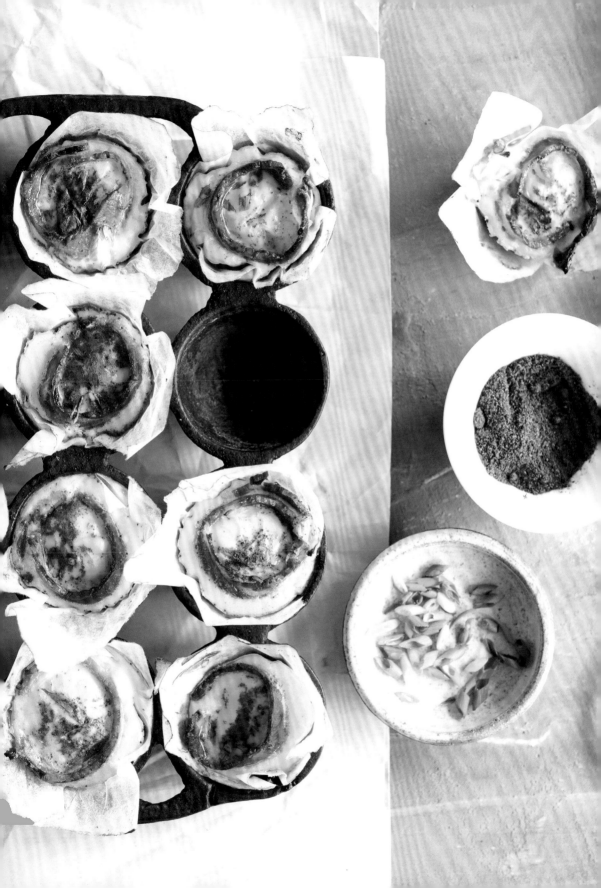

Cashew cream

1 cup (160g) raw cashews, pre-soaked

1 cup (250ml) filtered water

1 Medjool date, pitted

1. Place all ingredients in a powerful blender or food processor.

2. Blend on high until the nuts start to form a smooth paste. You may need to use a wooden spoon to stir the mixture occasionally, or even add water to reach the right consistency.

3. Store in an airtight container in the refrigerator for up to 3 days to use as a sweeter side for breakfasts or desserts.

Chai-spiced poached pears

—— SERVES 4 ——

3 cups (750ml) filtered water

1/2 cup (65g) frozen or fresh raspberries

2 tbsp loose leaf chai tea mix

3 tbsp red wine vinegar

3-4 small pears

Chopped pistachios, to serve

1. In a medium pot, bring the filtered water to the boil.

2. Add the raspberries, chai tea and vinegar and mix well.

3. Peel and core the pears and slice into halves or quarters.

4. Once the water is boiling, add pears to the mixture and reduce heat to a low simmer.

5. Simmer for 30-40 minutes over low heat and leave in pot to cool.

6. Serve with a dollop of cashew cream and chopped pistachios.

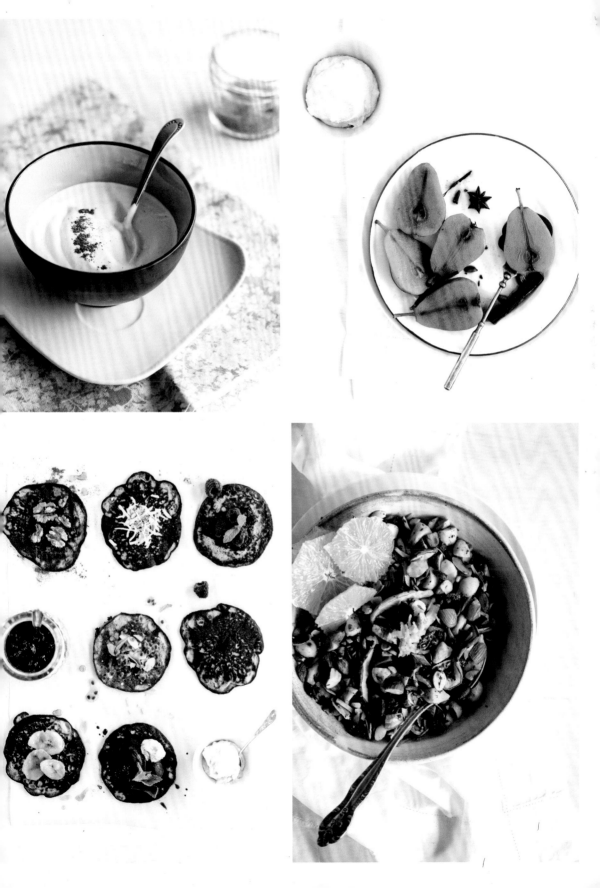

Holy-moly banana pancakes

1 banana

½ tsp ground cinnamon

½ tbsp almond butter

2 eggs

1 tbsp coconut oil

FOR THE TOPPING

½ cup (65g) frozen strawberries or berries of your choice

1 tsp balsamic vinegar

1. Put the banana, cinnamon, almond butter and eggs in a blender. Blend until well mixed and a little fluffy.

2. Place a large pan over medium heat and add the coconut oil. Once hot, slowly pour the pancake mixture into the pan (about 9cm/3 inches across). When bubbles start to form on the surface, flip the pancakes and cook through the second side.

3. For the topping, defrost the strawberries in the microwave for 30 seconds until soft (you can also do this in a pot if you prefer). Add the balsamic vinegar and mix well using the back of a fork. Topping should be sauce-like.

4. Serve with any toppings that you like!

Here are some creative pancake topping ideas: walnuts, maple bananas, cinnamon, raspberries, coconut flakes, passionfruit or cashew cream.

Clean mean muesli

1 cup (168g) raw almonds

1 cup (140g) natural macadamias

½ cup (60g) raw pistachios

½ cup (80g) raw cashews

2 cups (150g) organic, dried coconut chips (flakes)

½ cup (70g) pepitas (pumpkin seeds)

¼ cup (40g) chia seeds

1 tbsp ground cinnamon

1 tbsp ground fresh ginger

¼ cup (52g) coconut oil

1. Preheat the oven to 85°C/185°F. Low temperatures will help to avoid damaging the healthy nut oils and create crispier muesli.

2. Roughly chop all the nuts into chunky pieces.

3. Mix all the dry ingredients in a large bowl. Add the coconut oil and mix well.

4. Spread the muesli in a thin layer on a baking paper lined oven tray.

5. Bake for 15 minutes until crispy and starting to brown.

6. Let the muesli cool and store in an airtight container.

TIP: Serve muesli with homemade nut milk or sprinkle on top of smoothies.

Chorizo and chilli frittata

—— SERVES 4-6 ——

1 tsp coconut oil

1 high quality chorizo, sliced

1 garlic clove, crushed

½ hot red chilli, de-seeded and roughly chopped

½ white onion, diced

½ red capsicum (pepper), chopped

1 can (400g) chopped tomatoes

2 tbsp sliced Kalamata olives

8-12 eggs (depending on the size of your dish)

Fresh micro-greens, to serve

Handful of cherry tomatoes, to serve

Salt and pepper

1. Preheat the oven to 175°C/350°F and line a frittata tin with baking paper.

2. In a medium saucepan, heat the oil over a high heat. Add the sliced chorizo and pan fry until crispy and browned. Transfer to a plate and set aside.

3. In the same pan over medium heat add the garlic, chilli and onion and stir until translucent and soft.

4. Reduce to medium heat. Add the capsicum, olives and canned tomatoes and simmer for 15 minutes, stirring occasionally.

5. Into a large bowl, crack the eggs and whisk well.

6. Pour the eggs into the lined tin. Gently spoon the tomato mixture into the centre and use a fork to slowly stir the egg and sauce together using a circular motion. This will create a 'marbled' look when the frittata cooks.

7. Place in the oven for 10 minutes until the eggs start to cook. Remove from the oven and place the chorizo slices on top of the frittata. Put it back in the oven and bake until cooked through (another 5-10 minutes).

8. Garnish with micro-greens, cherry tomatoes and salt and pepper.

This recipe works for individual servings too. Follow the steps as above and spoon the mixture into a muffin tray or small frittata tins, simply adjust the cooking time accordingly.

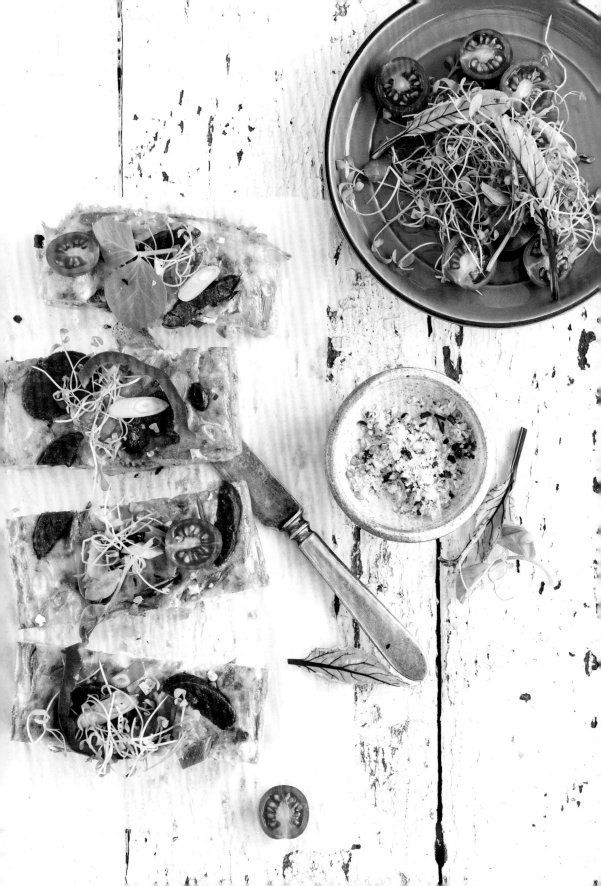

Sweet potato fritters

1 medium sweet potato
(400g/14oz)

1 egg

1 tsp salt

Ground black pepper, to
taste

1 tsp Moroccan seasoning
(check for hidden sugars)

2 tbsp coconut oil

1. Peel the sweet potato and grate using a food processor or cheese grater.

2. In a large bowl, crack the egg and whisk. Add the sweet potato, salt, pepper and Moroccan seasoning to the egg and mix well.

3. Heat the coconut oil over high heat and add the batter to fit as many fritters as possible in your pan (¼ cup or 3 tbsp at a time).

4. Fry for 2½ minutes on each side. The edges should start to brown and the fritter will hold together when you flip it.

5. When done, remove from the pan and serve warm. Fritters are a great replacement for toast, pancakes or on their own.

TIP: Once cooked, the fritters freeze well in an airtight container or bag. Pop them in the toaster to defrost on the spot!

These fritters are a fantastic transition food when you feel like toast or need something to hold up your eggs! They are delicious served with hard-boiled or poached eggs.

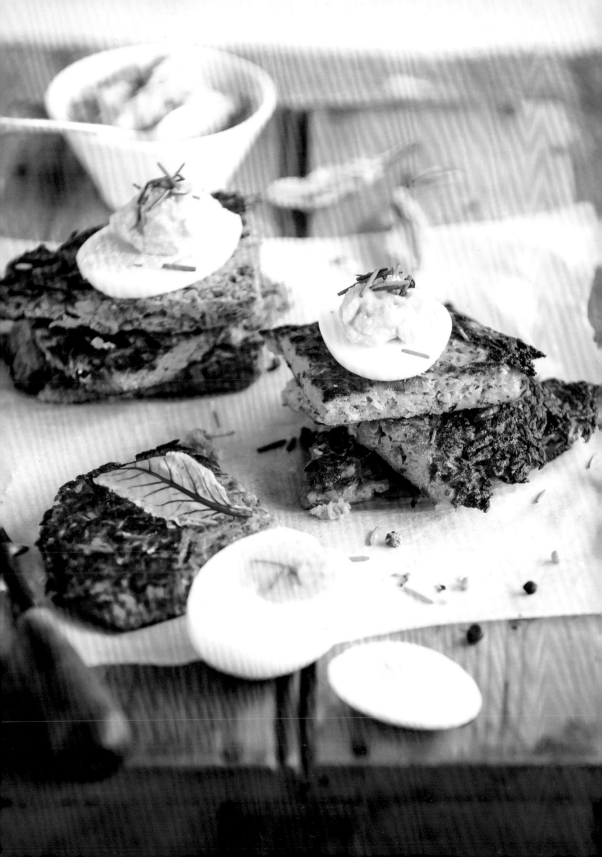

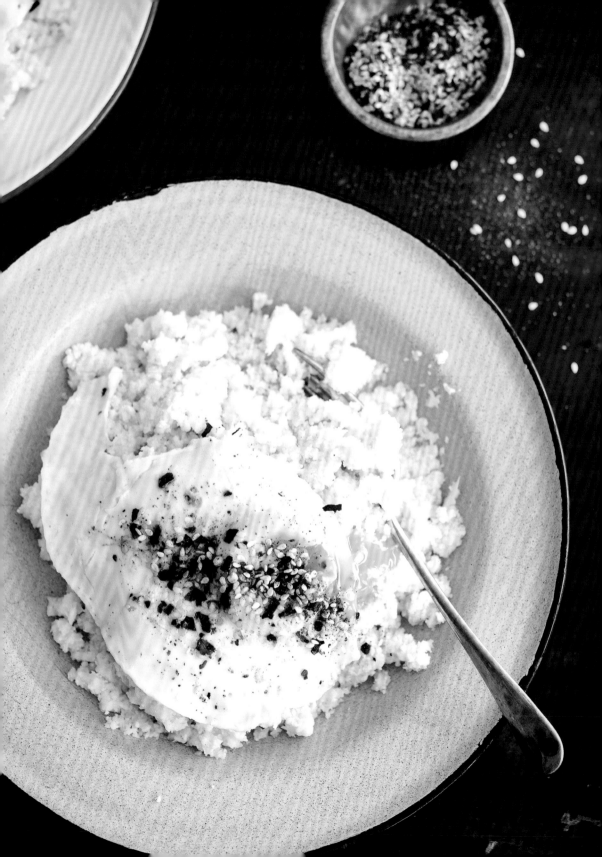

Spicy steam-fried eggs on cauliflower rice

—— SERVES 2 ——

This recipe uses a technique called steam frying. It's an easy, no-flip way to create a perfectly cooked fried egg without having to cross your fingers that the yolk won't break!

1 tsp smoked paprika

½ tsp sesame seeds

1 tsp chilli flakes (optional)

½ tsp salt

1 tsp ghee (or coconut oil)

4 eggs, at room temperature

1-2 tbsp water

1 cup cauliflower rice (page 80)

1. Mix the paprika, sesame seeds, chilli and salt in a small bowl.

2. Use a large fry pan with a glass lid and heat the ghee over high heat. Swirl it around to coat the pan.

3. Reduce to medium heat and gently crack the eggs into the pan. Sprinkle with the spice mix.

4. With the lid in one hand, pour the water into the hot pan and cover immediately.

5. The water will create steam that swirls up and over the eggs, cooking them from the top down.

6. As soon as the yolk becomes white in colour, remove the pan from the heat. The white should be cooked through and the yolk still runny.

7. Serve the eggs on top of salted cauliflower rice.

TIP: Create the flavour that you like by mixing up the seasonings. This recipe is also delicious when the spice blend is substituted for Moroccan or Cajun seasoning, or a pre-made Dukkah.

SNACKS

Capsicum dippers with guacamole boats
Capsicum and chilli sweet potato dip
Kale chips
Dijon devilled eggs
Clean zucchini slice
Apple slices with cashew cream
Sweet potato chips
Mama's mayo
Gathered trail mix

Capsicum dippers with guacamole boats

2 ripe Hass avocados (or other variety)

½ Spanish (red) onion (50g), peeled and finely diced

Juice from 1 lime

1 tsp freshly ground salt

1 tsp freshly ground pepper

1 small red chilli, diced (optional)

4 capsicums (peppers), one in each colour if possible!

1. Using a sharp knife, cut each avocado lengthways through to the seed. Using your hands, twist both halves in opposite directions as you pull the fruit apart.

2. Hack the seed with your knife and gently twist it out of the avocado.

3. Using a spoon, scoop all of the flesh into a bowl. Set the avocado skins aside for later.

4. Into the bowl with the avocado, add the diced onion, lime juice, salt, pepper and chilli.

5. Smash with the back of a fork until well mixed. Spoon the avocado mixture back into the avocado skins and serve with cold slices of rainbow capsicum.

Capsicum and chilli sweet potato dip

1 large sweet potato (about 400g/14oz)

1 tbsp coconut oil, melted

1 large red capsicum (pepper)

2 tbsp olive oil

1 tsp chilli flakes

1 tsp cumin

2 tsp smoked paprika

¼ cup (60ml) water

1 tbsp tahini (sesame seed paste)

juice of 2 lemons

Salt to taste

1. Preheat the oven to 180°C/356°F.

2. Peel the sweet potato and chop into small chunks. In a bowl, stir through the coconut oil to lightly coat all the pieces.

3. Roast in the oven for 35 minutes until soft.

4. Meanwhile, slice the red capsicum into about 6 pieces and place in an ovenproof dish. Roast for 10-15 minutes until soft.

5. Place the potato, red capsicum and all remaining ingredients into a powerful blender or food processor. Blend on high until smooth and creamy.

6. Store in a recycled jar or airtight container in the refrigerator for 4-5 days.

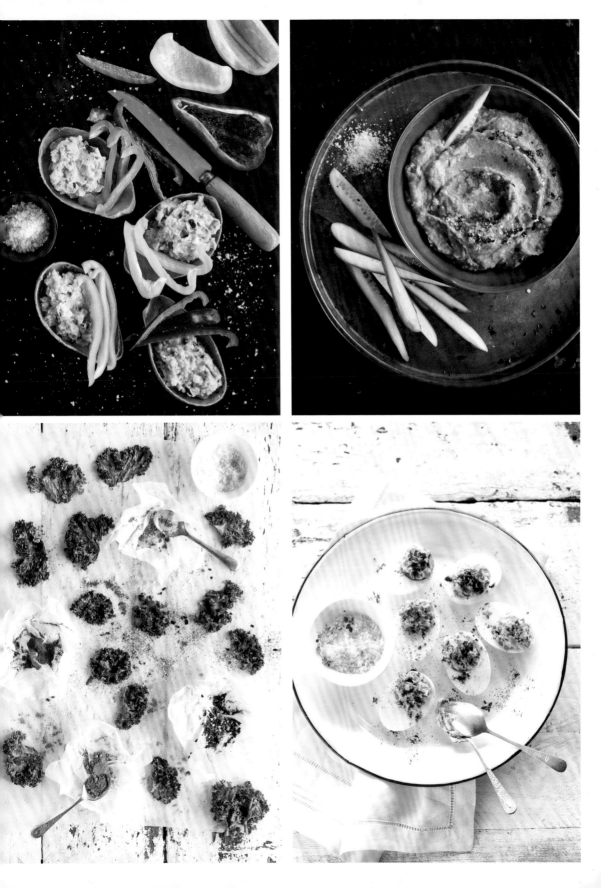

Kale Chips

— **SERVES 4-6** —

When transitioning to a cleaner diet, it is often difficult to find snack foods that hit the spot when you are looking for something salty and crunchy. These kale chips are super easy to make and can be seasoned in lots of different ways to mimic some of the snack foods that we're used to. Kale (also referred to as Tuscan cabbage) is an amazing power food. Per calorie, kale has more iron than beef and more calcium than milk, and is packed full of vitamins A, K and C, and antioxidants with cancer-fighting properties.

1 large bunch (700g/1.5lb) of kale (Tuscan cabbage), washed

2 tbsp (25g) melted coconut oil (or Ghee)

Salt to taste

1. Pre-heat the oven to 175°C/350°F and line a large tray with baking paper.

2. Remove the kale leaves from their fibrous stems with a knife or by tearing them off with your hands. Tear the leaves into bite-sized pieces.

3. In a mixing bowl, add the kale, coconut oil and salt and mix really well with your hands to coat the leaves.

4. Scatter onto the baking paper one layer thick.

5. Bake in the oven for 7-10 minutes, until the kale is still green in colour but crispy and dry. These paper-thin chips can burn very quickly so watch them closely in the last couple of minutes.

6. These will stay crispy in an airtight container for a couple of days.

TIP: Spice up the flavour of your kale chips by adding different spices and seasonings. Here are a few favourites to add to your chips before they go into the oven.

- French onion: ½ tbsp onion powder + 1 tsp garlic powder + 1 tsp salt
- Smoked chilli: ½ tbsp smoked paprika + 1 tsp chilli flakes
- Cheesy: 1 tbsp nutritional yeast + 1 tsp mustard powder
- Anti-inflam: 1 tbsp turmeric + 1 tsp ground ginger
- Spice: 1 tbsp cinnamon + dash of cayenne pepper

Dijon devilled eggs

—— SERVES 4 ——

These tasty little morsels are a great option for a pre-made quick breakfast or a snack high in protein and good fats. They'd be a great option for guests at brunch.

4 eggs

3 cups (750ml) water

1 tsp baking soda

4 slices (100g) high quality ham off the bone

1 tsp macadamia or coconut oil

1 tbsp Dijon-style mustard

1 tsp apple cider vinegar

Salt and pepper, to taste

1 tbsp paprika

1. Gently place the eggs in the bottom of a saucepan and add the water and baking soda. Make sure the water completely covers the eggs. Baking soda helps to separate the egg from the shell (making it easier to peel) by drawing some of the egg's water content out through the shell into the pot. Older eggs will also peel more easily, so choose eggs that are at least a week old to get dent free devilled egg baskets.

2. Heat the saucepan over high heat and when the water starts to boil, wait one minute before turning off the heat and covering the pot.

3. Leave the eggs for 10 minutes before dunking into ice water to arrest the cooking process.

4. Meanwhile, dice the ham and pan-fry with the oil until brown and crispy. Leave to cool.

5. Peel the eggs and slice in half lengthways. Scoop out the yolks into a separate bowl using a teaspoon.

6. Add the ham, mustard, vinegar, salt and pepper to the yolks and mix well to create a paste.

7. Using a teaspoon, evenly scoop the mustard mixture into the egg-white baskets.

8. Season each devilled egg with some paprika and a little salt.

TIP: For takeaway Dijon devils, press the two egg halves back together and store in an airtight container in the refrigerator.

Clean zucchini slice

⅔ cup (150g) bacon (look for one without nitrates or added sugar)

3-4 cups (600g) grated zucchini (about 3 medium sized)

2 small brown onions

8 eggs

1¼ cups (140g) raw almond meal

⅓ cup (75g) macadamia nut oil

1 small red chilli, finely diced

1. Preheat the oven to 175°C/350°F and line a 15 x 30 cm (6 x 12 inches) dish with baking paper.

2. Dice the bacon and fry over high heat until brown and crispy.

3. Meanwhile, wash and grate the zucchini and onions.

4. In a large mixing bowl, whisk the eggs and then stir through the almond meal.

5. Add the zucchini, onion, oil, chilli and pre-cooked bacon and mix well. The mixture should be just pourable.

6. Pour into the lined baking dish and bake for 40 minutes or until cooked through.

7. Leave to cool before slicing into small squares.

8. The slice should last in the refrigerator for 3-4 days and will freeze well too!

Skip the bacon for a vegetarian version. You can also add extra ingredients into this recipe depending on what you have available. It's delicious with sweet potato, chopped tomatoes and mushrooms.

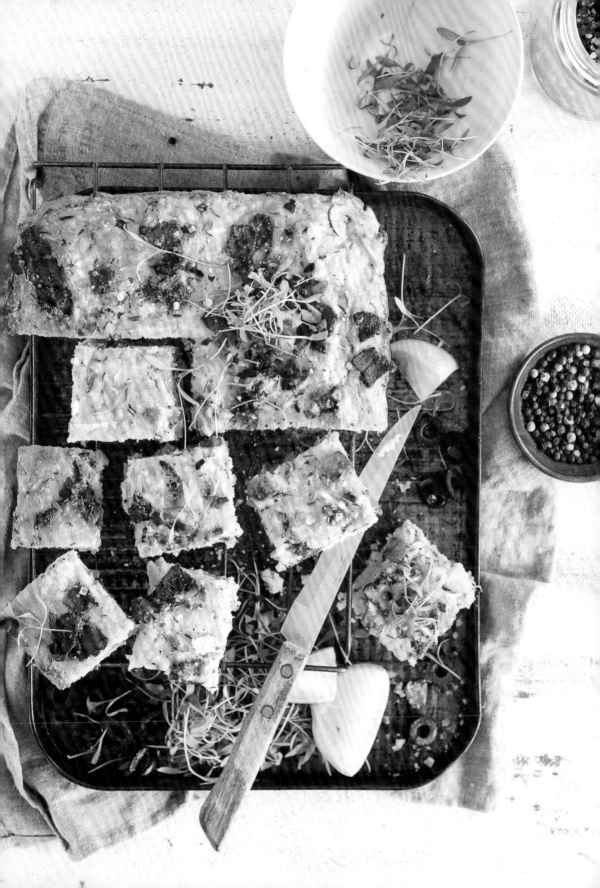

Apple slices with cashew cream

—— SERVES 2 ——

1 Granny Smith apple, washed

Juice from ½ lemon

2 cups (500ml) water

4 tbsp (60g) cashew cream (page 46)

Cinnamon to taste

1. Using a sharp knife, thinly slice the apple into flat discs.

2. Place the lemon juice and water in a bowl.

3. Dip the apple slices into the lemon water. This will stop them from oxidising and turning brown. If you're eating them straight away you can skip this step.

4. Spread a little cashew cream on each apple 'cracker' and season with a dash of cinnamon.

INGREDIENT SPOTLIGHT

Cinnamon is used as both a sweet and savoury spice and comes from the inner bark of several trees from the genus Cinnamomum. It's been shown to help to control blood sugar levels and has been used in studies with diabetic patients for this reason. To make use of this property, sprinkle cinnamon on sweeter foods like fruit and chocolate to balance the blood sugar response.

Sweet potato chips

—— SERVES 3-4 ——

Orange sweet potatoes are one of the best sources of beta-carotene. As carotenes are fat-soluble, make sure you enjoy them with some healthy fats to get the full benefit of this vitamin A precursor. This recipe pairs the sweet potato with coconut oil to help with nutrient absorption.

2 medium sweet potatoes (about 250g or 9oz each), very finely sliced

2 tbsp coconut oil, melted

salt, to taste

cinnamon (optional)

1. Preheat the oven to 175°C/350°F and line a large tray with baking paper.

2. In a large bowl, combine the sweet potato slices and coconut oil until all sides are lightly coated.

3. Lay the slices in a single layer on the baking paper. If you have extra potatoes, use a second tray or cook two batches.

4. Place in the oven and bake for 10 minutes on each side (watch closely as they burn quickly)

5. To bring out the flavour of the sweet potato, sprinkle with salt and cinnamon to taste.

6. These are best served straight out of the oven!

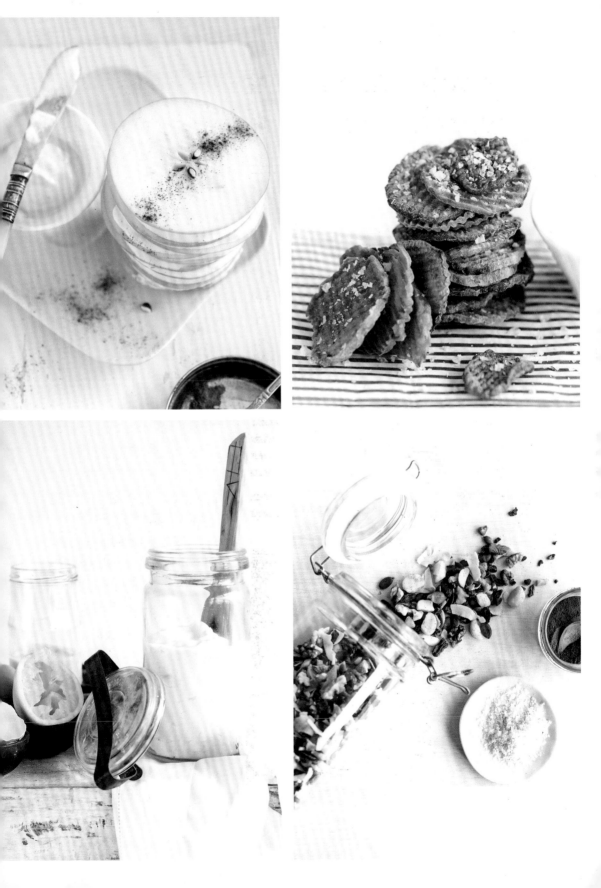

Mama's mayo

There are lots of Paleo mayonnaise variations that use high quality oils instead of rancid vegetable oils and preservatives that you'll find lurking in supermarket varieties. Although we'd usually recommend an extra virgin, cold-pressed olive oil, this recipe calls for a light flavoured olive oil as we found that other oils were quite overpowering compared to the mayo that we're used to.

1 egg, at room temperature

2 tbsp apple cider vinegar or lemon juice

½ tsp Dijon-style mustard (or dry mustard powder)

½ tsp salt

¼ tsp cayenne pepper (optional)

1¼ cups (310ml) extra light tasting olive oil

1. In a food processor (or blender), add the egg, vinegar, mustard, salt, cayenne pepper and ¼ cup of the light olive oil.

2. Process until just combined.

3. Place the remaining cup of olive oil in a small jug with a good pouring spout.

4. With your food processor or blender churning on medium, pour in the olive oil in a very slow, steady stream. Do not rush this process.

5. After a few minutes of pouring, you'll hear the food processor change notes as the consistency of the mayo changes. This happens when the oil starts to form an emulsion with the egg and mustard.

6. Continue to slowly add the rest of the oil. You'll end up with a mayonnaise that will hold its own shape and form the consistency that we're used to.

7. Transfer to a recycled jar and store in the refrigerator for up to a week.

TIP: For herbed mayo, stir in a ¼ cup (5g) chopped fresh herbs like dill, coriander or parsley.

Gathered trail mix

—— **SERVES 10** ——

This mix is an excellent afternoon pick-me-up snack that beats a processed option like potato chips or a chocolate bar. Be prepared and keep a small container in your bag or at your desk so you can nibble on good quality fats and loads of minerals when you feel like a snack.

1 cup (75g) coconut flakes (you can buy these dehydrated or dry roast them in a pan for a couple of minutes to make them crunchy)

¾ cup (105g) macadamia nuts, roughly chopped

½ cup (130g) walnuts, roughly chopped

½ cup (50g) goji berries

½ cup (60g) raw cacao nibs

2 tsp cinnamon

1 tsp Himalayan rock salt

½ cup (70g) pepitas (pumpkin seeds)

1. Combine all ingredients in a mixing bowl. Keep in an airtight container or divide into servings for a snack on the run or lunch box filler.

INGREDIENT SPOTLIGHT

Cacao nibs are small chunks of cacao beans that have been cultivated in South America and Mexico for thousands of years. Cacao beans have been used as a currency in some cultures — the Aztecs even believed them to be of divine origin! Cacao is a form of chocolate that has not been combined with sugar, milk solids and other industrial ingredients, and is full of nutrients. It is one of the best sources of Magnesium, which balances brain chemistry, builds strong bones, and helps regulate heartbeat and blood pressure. Magnesium is also believed to play a role in preventing muscle cramps and improved recovery for active people.

SALADS
AND SIDES

Roast beetroot and baby broccoli salad with toasted seeds

Sweet potato salad

Primal party platter

Maple roasted carrots

Cabbage, coriander and carrot salad with sesame vinaigrette

Brussels, bacon and butter

Toasted seeds

Emergency kale

Classic herb roast vegetables

Cauliflower 3 ways

Spicy pumpkin and coconut soup

Padma's pumpkin curry

Tuna Nicoise salad

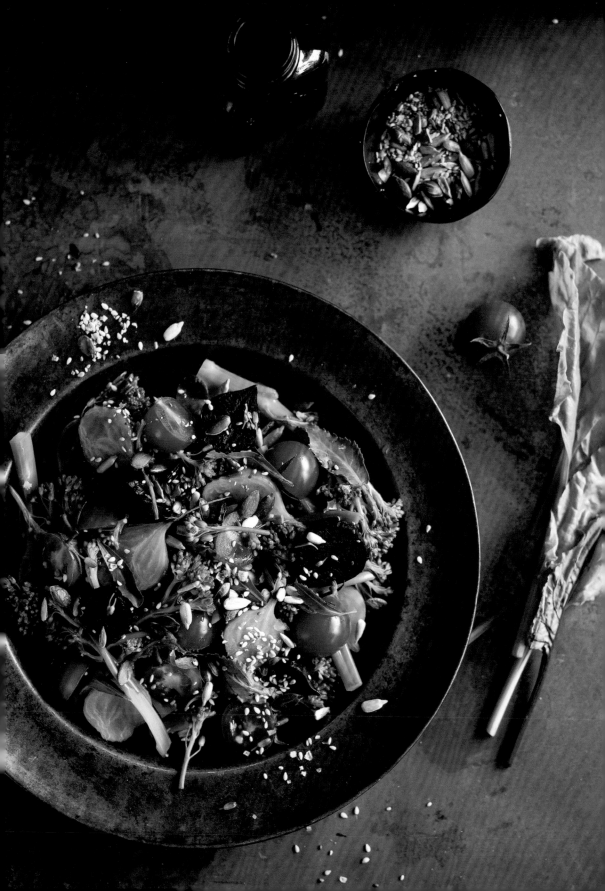

Roast beetroot and baby broccoli salad with toasted seeds

2 whole beetroot

1 bunch baby broccoli

1 tbsp ghee, melted

1 tbsp balsamic vinegar

8 cherry tomatoes, sliced

1 tbsp olive oil

2 tbsp toasted seeds
(page 75)

1. Preheat the oven to 175°C/350°F.

2. Bring a small pot of water to the boil.

3. Wash the beetroot and chop off both ends. Par-boil for 10 minutes.

4. Meanwhile, wash the broccoli well and chop the bunch in half.

5. Carefully remove the beetroot from the pot and peel while running it under cold water. This will help to prevent the colour from staining your hands and bench top.

6. Cut the beetroot into small pieces and add to a bowl with the melted ghee and balsamic vinegar. Mix well and then spread onto a tray lined with baking paper.

7. Bake the beetroot for about 30 minutes, or until chewy and cooked through.

8. Meanwhile, drop the broccoli into a pot of boiling water and blanche for 3 minutes. Remove and dunk straight into iced water to keep it crisp and bright green.

9. Combine the broccoli, beetroot, cherry tomatoes and a dash of olive oil. Top with the lightly toasted seeds to serve.

A little feta is a delicious addition to this salad too.

Sweet potato salad

This is a much healthier take on the classic potato salad recipe. By using sweet potato, we're getting access to higher levels of beta-carotene and more nutritional value.

4 cups (1 litre) water

3 large orange sweet potatoes

4 eggs, hard-boiled

¼ cup (60ml) apple cider vinegar

¼ cup (60g) Dijon-style mustard

½ cup (125ml) macadamia nut oil (or extra virgin olive oil)

1 tbsp sesame oil

2 tbsp fresh chives, chopped

Salt and pepper to taste

1. Bring a pot of water to the boil.

2. Peel and chop the sweet potato into bite-sized chunks and add to the water to cook for 10 minutes or until the potato starts to soften. Once cooked, drain and sprinkle with salt and pepper. Let cool.

3. Peel the hard-boiled eggs and cut in half. Remove the yolks, break them up with a fork and set aside. Roughly chop the egg whites.

4. In a large pitcher or mixing bowl make the dressing by combining the vinegar, mustard, salt and pepper, egg whites and egg yolks.

5. Whisk the dressing and slowly add the macadamia nut oil and sesame oil. Continue to whisk until the liquid forms an emulsion (combines together).

6. In a large bowl, fold the dressing and chopped fresh chives through the sweet potato chunks. Be gentle so that it doesn't turn into a mash. Garnish with extra chives.

7. Leave to marinate in the refrigerator for a few hours or overnight.

This is a great salad to bring along to your next barbecue and is always very popular!

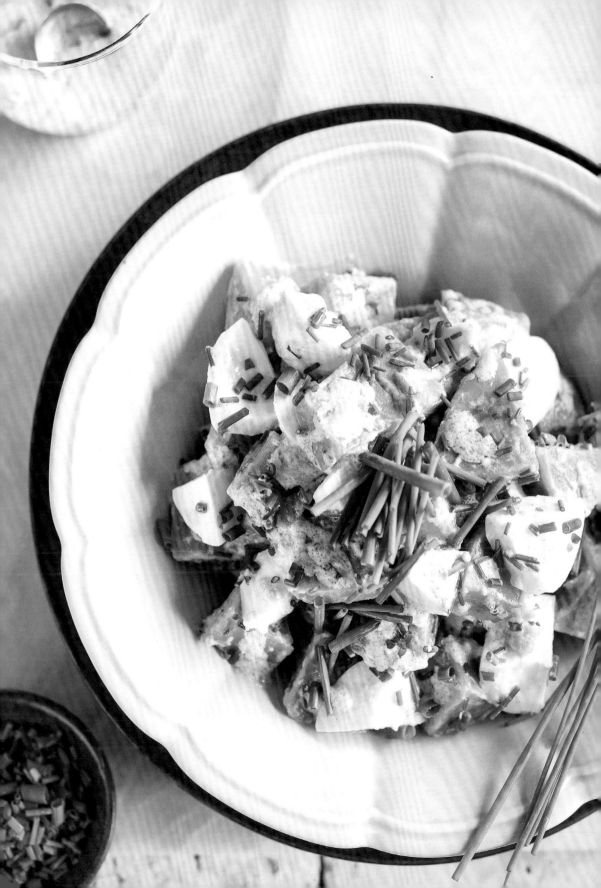

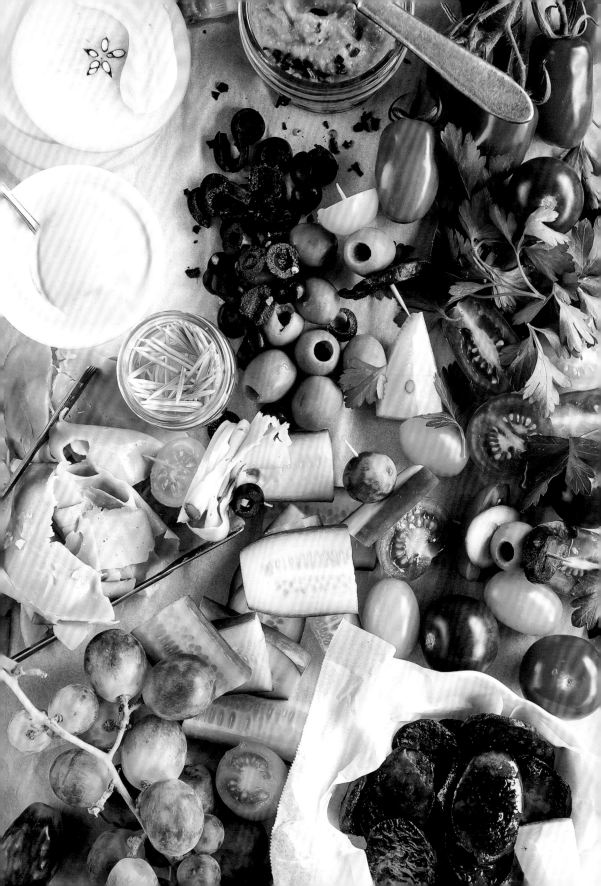

Primal party platter

This party platter will satisfy your guests and they won't even realise that it doesn't have crackers and cheese!

1 tsp coconut oil or ghee

1 Spanish chorizo

2 Granny Smith apples, sliced thinly

mixed cherry tomatoes, try to get different colours

6-8 slices (200g) ham (nitrate free)

½ cup (90g) mixed olives

1 small cucumber, sliced

½ cup (120g) cashew cream (page 46)

½ cup (120g) capsicum and chilli sweet potato dip (page 58)

1. In a hot pan, melt the coconut oil.

2. Slice the chorizo into diagonal pieces and pan-fry until brown and crispy (about 5 minutes). Set aside to cool.

3. Arrange all ingredients on a serving platter and serve with toothpicks. Encourage combos like apple, chorizo and cashew cream or cucumber and dip wrapped in ham!

This platter can be adapted to suit the foods that you have available. Other ideas could include sauerkraut, pineapple, vegetable chips, nuts, veggies sticks and other healthy dips.

Maple roasted carrots

— SERVES 4 —

1 bunch of baby carrots with tops intact

3cm (3 tbsp) chunk of fresh ginger, peeled and grated

1½ tbsp ghee, melted

1 tbsp pure maple syrup

1. Preheat the oven to 150°C/300°F.

2. Chop the tops off the baby carrots, leaving about 6cm (2.36 inches) of the stem. Discard the tops.

3. Place carrots in a baking dish with the ghee, maple syrup and ginger. Mix well.

4. Roast for 10-15 minutes, until the carrots are starting to caramelise. You may need to stir them occasionally to prevent burning.

5. Serve as a sweeter side with roast chicken, steak or on their own.

INGREDIENT SPOTLIGHT

Maple syrup is one of the best sweetener options on a Paleo diet. Maple syrup is a natural product, a sweet sap created by the Maple tree. Compared to sweeteners like agave syrup and high fructose corn syrup, maple syrup has a much lower level of fructose and like raw honey, stevia and molasses, is much less processed and has been made for hundreds of years. Make sure that you buy a raw, real maple syrup in its natural form.

Cabbage, coriander and carrot salad with sesame vinaigrette

— SERVES 4 —

2 carrots, peeled and grated

½ head red cabbage, sliced finely

1 tbsp sesame seeds

½ cup (10g) fresh coriander leaves

¼ cup (60ml) extra virgin olive oil

1 tbsp lime juice

1 tsp apple cider vinegar

2 tsp sesame oil

1. In a large bowl, toss the grated carrot, cabbage, sesame seeds and coriander.

2. Measure all other ingredients into a glass jar. Screw the lid on tight and shake the jar until the mixture starts to bind together (emulsify).

3. Pour over salad and mix well.

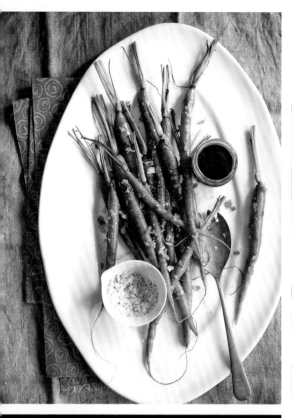

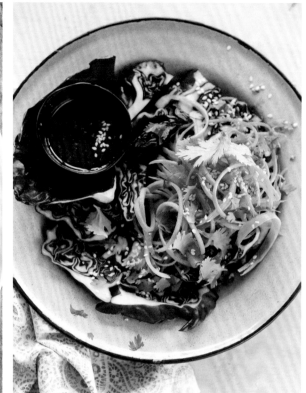

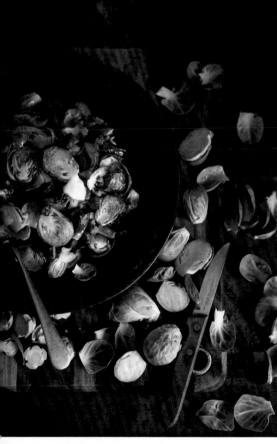

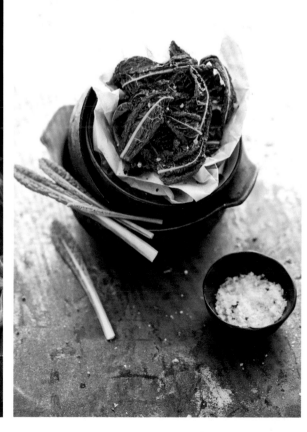

Brussels, bacon and butter

—— **SERVES 6** ——

To optimise nutrient absorption of vegetables, it's important to eat them with some healthy fats. This salty and crispy combo will win over even the most stubborn disapprovers!

4 cups (400g) Brussels sprouts

3 tbsp ghee, melted

1 brown onion, diced

3 slices (75g) bacon (nitrate free), diced

1 tsp salt

1. Preheat the oven to 200°C/390°F. Line a large baking tray with aluminium foil.

2. In a large pan, add 1 tbsp of the ghee, diced onion and bacon. Pan-fry for about 5 minutes, stirring frequently.

3. Wash the Brussels sprouts and remove any damaged or loose leaves. Chop off the stalk and cut in half lengthways.

4. Place the Brussels sprouts in the baking tray with the remaining ghee, bacon, onion and salt. Roast for 45-50 minutes, stirring occasionally.

5. The Brussels sprouts should be tender and starting to brown.

6. This dish is best eaten straight away, as Brussels sprouts can go bitter if left to sit.

INGREDIENT SPOTLIGHT

Brussels sprouts contain sulforaphane, a chemical with potent anticancer properties. They are also believed to boost DNA repair in cells and just one and a half cups of Brussels sprouts contains about 430 milligrams of omega-3 fatty acids (about 1/3 of the daily recommended amount). They also contain a high level of vitamin K, which helps to regulate anti-inflammatory responses.

Toasted seeds

This toasted seed mix adds some healthy fats and crunchy texture to almost any salad. Pre-make a big batch and store in an airtight jar in your pantry. The trick in making this mix is to make sure that the temperature of the pan is kept as low as possible to avoid damaging the unsaturated seed oils.

½ cup (77g) sesame seeds

½ cup (70g) pepitas (pumpkin seeds)

½ cup (70g) sunflower seeds

2 tbsp chia seeds

2 tsp salt flakes

1. Into a large dry pan on *low* heat, add the sunflower seeds and pepitas. Using a wooden spoon or spatula, stir the seeds constantly to make sure they don't burn. Mix well for about 60 seconds.

2. Add the sesame seeds and stir for another minute, or until all seeds are a light toasted brown.

3. Transfer to a bowl and set aside until cool. Add the chia seeds and salt and mix well.

4. Store in a recycled jar in a cool, dark place.

Emergency kale

This is a quick, easy and very nutritious vegetable option when you get caught out and need to get some greens on the table, fast. It's delicious under a couple fried eggs for breakfast, or as a side with dinner. It's a great idea to whip up a big batch and store in the refrigerator for fast meals and lunch building.

2 tbsp coconut oil

1 big bunch of curly kale (Tuscan cabbage), washed and chopped finely

2 tsp Cajun spice (without sugar)

Salt, to taste

1. In a large pan, heat the coconut oil on high.

2. Add the chopped kale. It should crackle a little when it hits the hot pan.

3. Add the seasoning and stir frequently for about 3 minutes as the kale cooks through and starts to brown.

Classic herb roast vegetables

Particularly in winter, a big batch of roast veggies is a great side for any meat dish or as a real-food option for post training recovery. You can make a big batch of these to have on hand for lunches and high carbohydrate snacks.

½ (1.5kg/3.3lb) Kent pumpkin, or other variety

4 small Spanish (red) onions, peeled

4 (1.5 kg/3.3lb) large sweet potatoes, peeled

3 (20g) garlic cloves, peeled

3 tbsp ghee, melted

¼ cup (8g) chopped fresh rosemary

2 tbsp fresh lemon thyme

2 tsp ground salt flakes

1. Preheat the oven to 200°C/390°F. Line a large baking dish with aluminium foil to make clean-up easier.

2. Using a sharp knife, remove most of the pumpkin skin, but not all.

3. Chop the pumpkin, onion and sweet potato into large chunks and place them in the baking dish. Drizzle with the ghee and mix well.

4. In a small bowl, combine the salt, rosemary and thyme. Sprinkle over the veggies.

5. Roast for 75 minutes, turning once, or until tender and lightly golden.

A touch of balsamic vinegar can be a great addition to roast veggies as they're cooking and will create and rustic glaze and add a deep red colour to the dish.

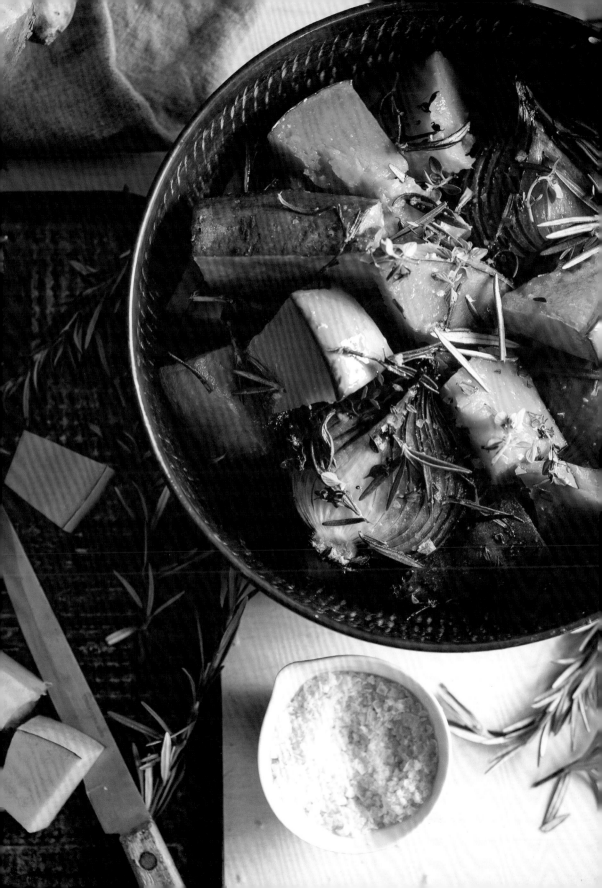

Cauliflower three ways

Cauliflower is a super-vegetable. It's jam packed with anti-inflammatory and cancer-fighting properties and is incredibly easy to whip up into a filling base for any meal. Cauliflower is a great way to sneak some veggies into your day or onto the plate of little ones! These are just three of the many ways that you can transform the humble cauliflower in your kitchen.

Cauliflower mash

—— **SERVES 8** ——

3 cups (750ml) water

1 large head of cauliflower, cut into chunks

2 tbsp ghee (or butter)

1 tsp salt

1 tbsp onion powder

1. Add the water to a large pot and bring to the boil.

2. Place the cauliflower chunks in a vegetable steamer and cover with the lid.

3. Steam over the pot of boiling water for 10 minutes or until the cauliflower is soft and cooked through.

4. Drain the cauliflower and add to a large bowl on your food processor, fitted with a standard chopping blade. A hand-held stick blender will work too.

5. Add the ghee, salt and onion powder.

6. Pulse until smooth. You may need to use a wooden spatula to stir the mixture once or twice.

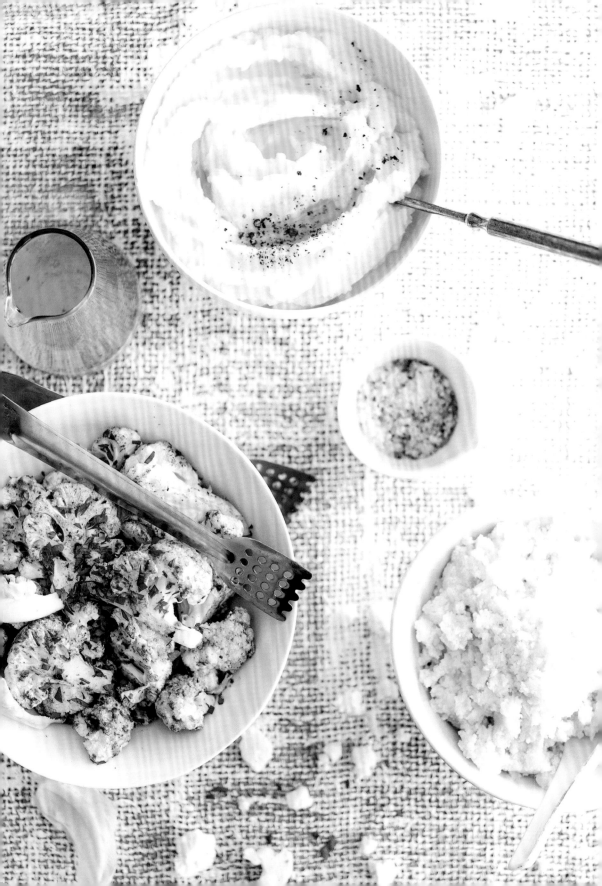

Cauliflower 'rice'

1 large head of cauliflower,
cut into chunks

2 tbsp ghee

1 tsp salt

1 tsp ground pepper

1. Put the raw cauliflower in the large bowl fitting of a food processor with a standard chopping blade. If you don't have one, you can finely dice the cauliflower with a sharp knife – it will just take a lot longer!

2. Pulse until the cauliflower pieces resemble rice grains. Be careful not to over-process, larger pieces are better than mush!

3. Heat the ghee in a large fry-pan on high.

4. Add the cauliflower 'rice' and salt and pepper.

5. Stir constantly for about 4 minutes with a wooden spoon as the rice cooks and starts to brown.

Coconut roasted cauliflower

1 large head of cauliflower

½ cup (125ml) coconut cream

1 tbsp cumin

2 tsp curry powder

1 tsp garlic powder

1 tsp chilli powder (optional)

1 tsp salt

Zest and juice of 1 lime

1. Preheat the oven to 200°C/390°F and line a large tray with baking paper.

2. Chop the cauliflower into large slices of a similar thickness and lay flat on the baking tray.

3. Combine all remaining ingredients in a small bowl.

4. Using a basting brush, coat the top of the cauliflower in the coconut-spice mixture.

5. Roast for 30 minutes. The coconut cream should make a 'crust' on the surface of the cauliflower.

6. This is a delicious base for Padma's pumpkin curry (page 89).

You can create all sorts of vegetable mashes and purees to complement most protein options. Examples include carrot and cauliflower puree, sweet potato mash, eggplant puree and chopped kale.

Spicy pumpkin and coconut soup

1 brown onion, diced

1 fresh red chilli (or 1 tsp chilli flakes)

1cm (1 tbsp) fresh ginger, finely grated

1 tbsp Ras El Hanout (Moroccan spice blend)

1 (7g) garlic clove, crushed

1 tbsp coconut oil

4 cups (900g/2lb) pumpkin, skin removed and flesh chopped

4 cups (1 litre) vegetable stock

½ can (200ml/6.8 fl oz) coconut cream (optional)

4-6 kaffir lime leaves, de-stemmed and thinly sliced

1. In a large saucepan over medium heat, fry the onion, chilli, ginger, lime leaves, Moroccan spices and garlic in the coconut oil for 2 minutes or until onion is soft.

2. Add the pumpkin and stir through for 1 minute.

3. Add the vegetable stock and bring to the boil.

4. Reduce to a simmer and cook for 20 minutes or until pumpkin is soft.

5. Once cooled a little, pulse the soup with a hand-stick mixer or in batches in a blender until smooth and creamy.

6. Return the soup to the pot, add the coconut cream (optional) and stir through until just mixed.

7. Serve topped with chilli flakes and kaffir lime leaves.

If you prefer a lighter soup, omit the coconut cream.

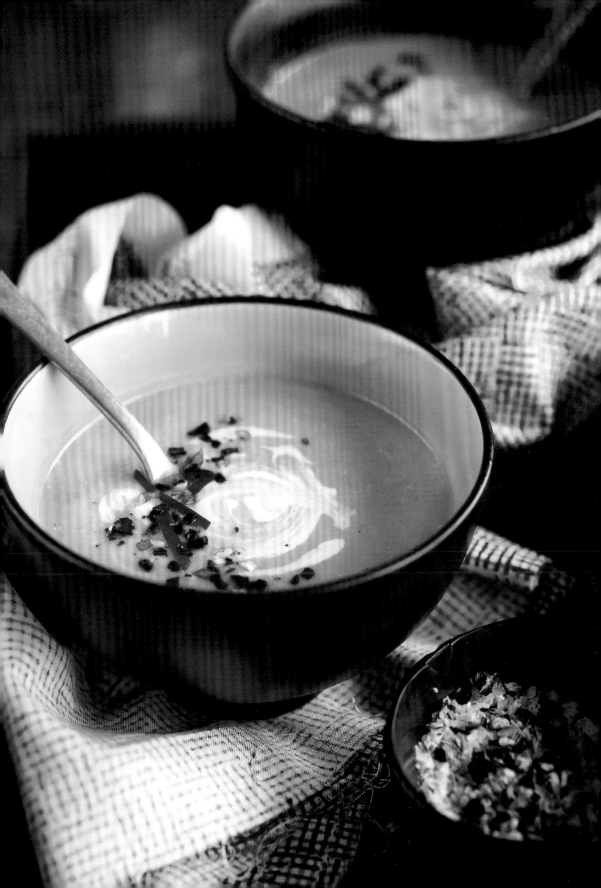

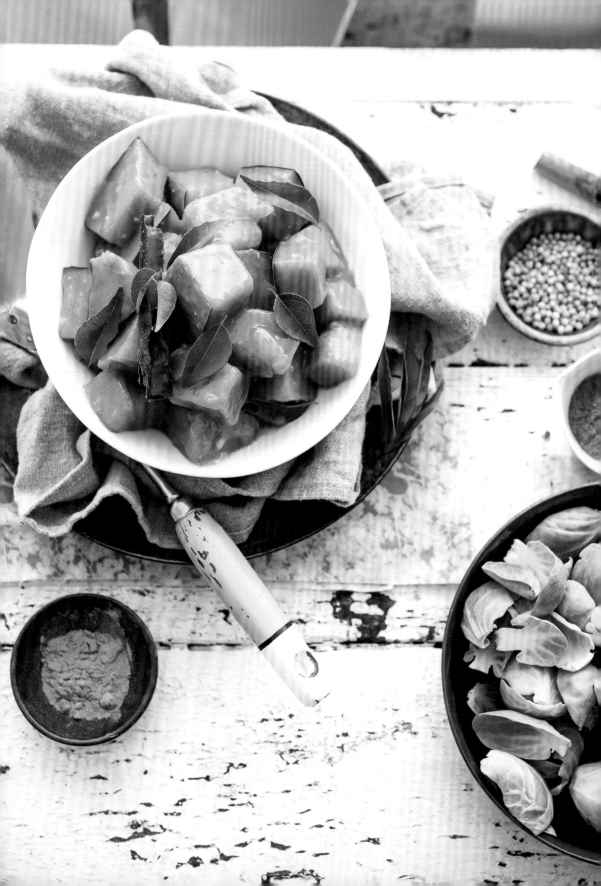

Padma's pumpkin curry

—— SERVES 8 ——

This Sri Lankan pumpkin curry recipe is an authentic and powerful blend of spices. It's one of the best ways to use up some extra pumpkin and is great on its own or as a creamy base for chicken or fish. The secret to this recipe is the weird and wonderful list of spices. Look out for a Sri Lankan grocery in your area, or jump online to find them. It's worth it!

¼ pumpkin, Kent variety is best

½ brown onion, diced

1-2 small green chillies, sliced

2-3 garlic cloves, sliced

2 curry leaves, roughly torn

½ tsp fenugreek seeds

½ cinnamon stick, crumbled

1 tsp Sri Lankan chilli powder

1 tsp curry powder (usually consists of ground coriander seeds, cumin and fennel)

⅛ tsp ground turmeric

1½ tsp salt

3-4 cups (750ml-1 litre) water

5 tbsp coconut powder

1. Take some of the outer skin off the pumpkin (but not all of it) then cut the pumpkin into 3cm (1 inch) cubes and place into a saucepan.

2. Add all other ingredients, except the coconut powder, and mix well.

3. Add enough water (3-4 cups) to nearly cover the pumpkin and boil for 5 minutes.

4. Add the coconut powder and mix thoroughly.

5. Leave to cook uncovered for 3-4 minutes until the liquid reduces and the pumpkin is creamy and tender.

6. Serve with cauliflower rice and green vegetables.

TIP: If you don't have coconut powder, substitute half of the water for coconut cream and add this when you boil the pumpkin.

Tuna Nicoise Salad

—— **SERVES 4** ——

The correct ingredients and presentation for an authentic French Nicoise salad are much debated. This version of a tuna Nicoise is all about building blocks for dinner parties, fast meals and pre-made lunches. You can pre-prepare all of the ingredients and then serve as a rainbow platter for a filling and high protein plate. If there's always a back-up can of tuna in your pantry, you can make this salad from whatever vegetables you have in the refrigerator!

1 tbsp red wine vinegar

¼ cup (60ml) cold-pressed olive oil

1 tsp Dijon-style mustard

2 large cans (350g/12oz) of tuna in spring water, drained*

½ Spanish (red) onion, diced

1 small cucumber, sliced

10 cherry tomatoes, halved

4 tbsp sauerkraut or other fermented vegetables

1 red capsicum (pepper), sliced

½ cup (10g) chopped fresh parsley

2 eggs, hard-boiled

*You can also use fresh tuna steaks, just marinade in a little macadamia nut oil for an hour. Heat a large skillet on medium high heat or place on a hot grill. Cook the steaks 2- 3 minutes on each side until cooked through.

1. Add the vinegar, olive oil and mustard into a glass jar with a screw top lid. Shake vigorously until well mixed and emulsified.

2. Arrange all salad ingredients around a large, flat bowl. Top with slices of hard-boiled egg.

3. Pour the vinaigrette over the salad and serve!

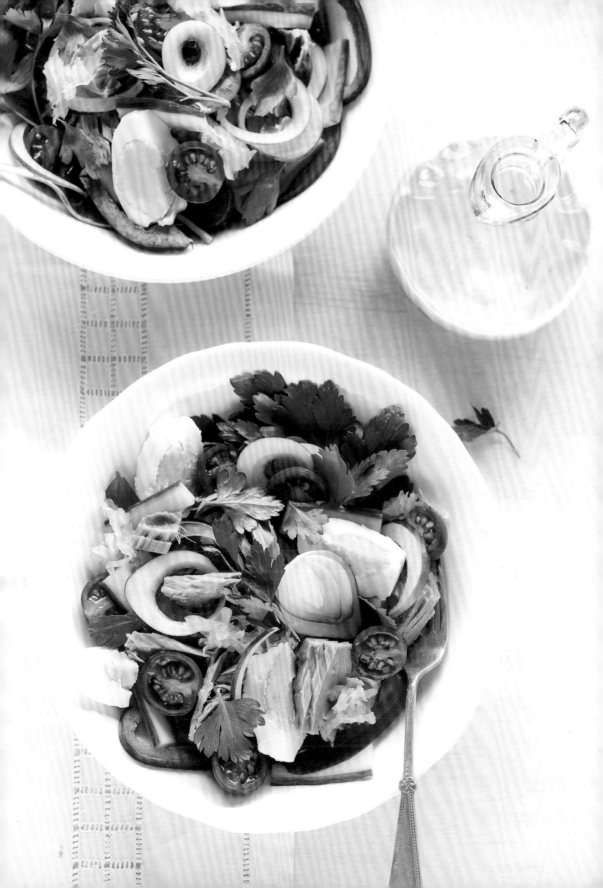

FISH,
POULTRY
AND MEAT

Macadamia and coconut crusted fish

Chicken san choy bow

Apricot chicken

Mini Sheppard's pie pots

Chermoula fish tacos

Sticky apple pork ribs

Chunky chilli con carne

Ginger chilli chicken

Chicken and kale pesto 'pasta'

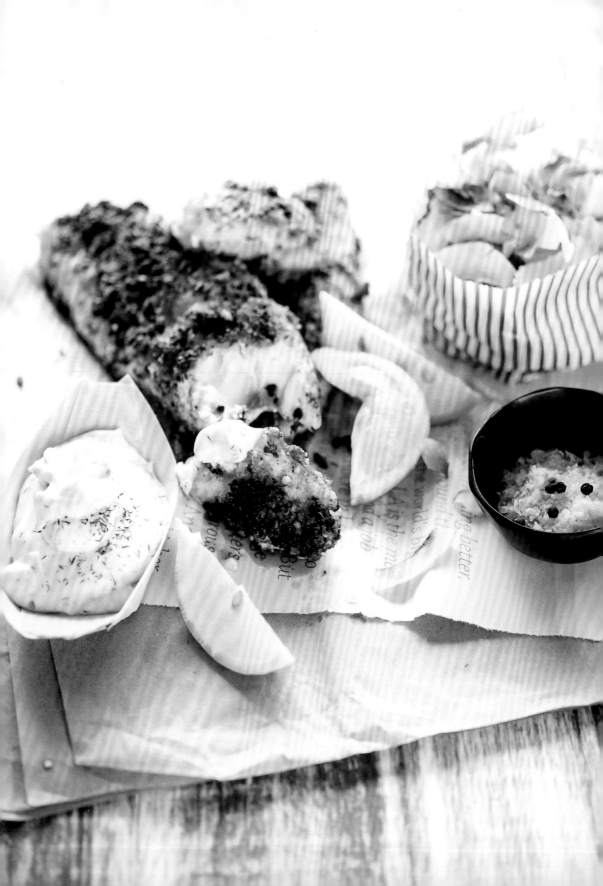

Macadamia and coconut crusted fish

250g (9oz) fresh white fish fillets (e.g. flathead tails)

½ cup (70g) raw macadamia nuts

½ cup (40g) desiccated coconut

½ tsp salt

½ tsp pepper

2 egg whites

4 tbsp coconut oil

½ cup (120g) mama's mayo (page 66) mixed with 2 tbsp lemon juice

1. Cut the fish into small strips of a similar size and thickness. Set aside.

2. In a food processor, grind the macadamia nuts into a course crumble. Add desiccated coconut, salt and pepper and mix well. Set aside in a wide-mouthed bowl or on a plate.

3. In a separate bowl, whisk the two egg whites and set aside.

4. Prepare all the fish pieces by firstly dipping them completely in the egg, then covering them with the macadamia and coconut mixture. Set aside on a separate plate.

5. In a medium-high pan, add the coconut oil and leave to heat up for 30 seconds. It should sizzle when you drop a piece of crumb in!

6. Fry each fish piece for 4 minutes on each side or until cooked to your liking.

7. Serve with lemon wedges and lemon-infused mayo.

The macadamia and coconut mixture is high in fats, so it will cook quite quickly and is easy to burn. Make sure the temperature of your pan isn't too high to ensure that the fish is cooked in the middle.

Chicken san choy bow

2 tbsp coconut oil, melted

1 brown onion, diced

2 garlic cloves, crushed

10-12 large iceberg lettuce leaves

500g (1.1lb) chicken mince

1 tbsp fresh ginger, grated

¼ tsp ground chilli

½ tsp cinnamon

1 tbsp sesame oil

¼ cup (60ml) coconut aminos or tamari

1 tbsp white wine vinegar

1 tbsp fresh lime juice

1 yellow capsicum (pepper), diced

1 green capsicum (pepper), diced

1 carrot, diced

Fresh sprouts to serve, e.g. snow pea sprouts

Mint leaves, to serve

1. In a pan, heat the coconut oil on high and add the onion and garlic. Cook for a few minutes until onion is translucent. Meanwhile, pop the lettuce leaves in some iced water to crisp up.

2. Add the chicken mince to the pan and use a spatula or spoon to break it up so there are no lumps. Add the ginger, chilli, cinnamon and sesame oil. Mix well to coat chicken and cook over medium heat for 3 minutes.

3. Add the coconut aminos, vinegar, lime juice and vegetables. Mix well and reduce heat to a simmer. Cover with a lid and cook for 3 more minutes.

4. Test the chicken to make sure it's cooked through but not dry. Adjust your chilli here to give it the kick you're after.

5. Serve the chicken mixture in small bowls with 2-3 lettuce cups per person. Garnish with sprouts, mint and lime wedges.

The chicken mince can be substituted for lamb, beef, pork or even kangaroo.

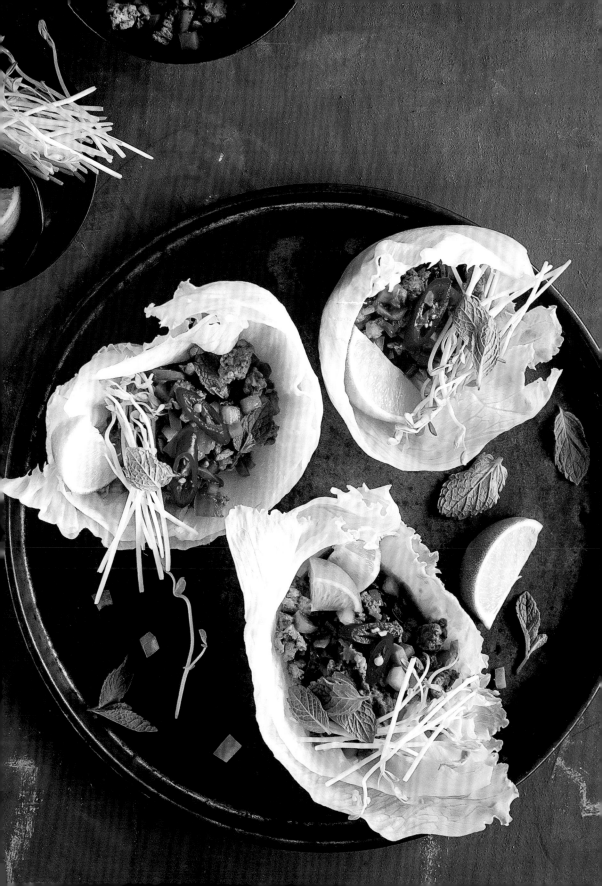

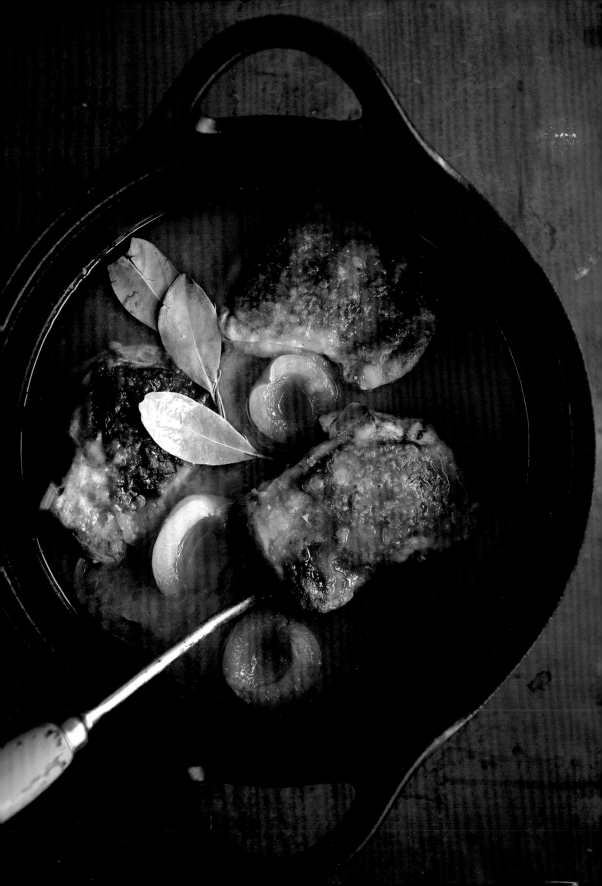

Apricot chicken

Here's a healthy take on this classic one-pot meal. No onion soup packets or sugary apricot syrup, but a whole lot of flavour!

2 tbsp macadamia nut oil

2 brown onions, cut into chunks

3 garlic cloves, crushed

600g (1.3lb) chicken thigh fillets, with skin

800g (1.8lb) canned apricots (sugar and preservative free) or 1kg (2.2lb) of fresh apricots, halved and pitted

1 tbsp Moroccan seasoning (sugar-free)

2 cups (500ml) vegetable or chicken stock

2-3 bay leaves

1 tsp sea salt

1. Preheat the oven to 180°C/355°F.

2. In a large cast iron pot or pan over medium-high heat, add the oil and chopped onions and garlic. Stir to soften.

3. If needed, add a little more oil then throw in the chicken thigh fillets. Brown the chicken for 2 minutes on each side.

4. Meanwhile, add one can of apricots to a blender with the Moroccan seasoning. Whizz until smooth. If you don't have a blender, you can mash the apricots in a bowl with a fork.

5. Once the chicken and onion have browned, add the blended apricots and reduce the heat. Stir the pot well.

6. Add the vegetable stock, bay leaves, second can of apricots and salt to the pot.

7. Place the casserole dish in the oven (with the lid on) or transfer to an ovenproof baking dish and cover with aluminium foil.

8. Bake for 60 minutes covered then remove lid or foil and return to the oven for another 10 minutes. The chicken should be tender and starting to fall apart.

9. Serve with cauliflower rice (page 84) or on its own.

Mini Sheppard's pie pots

—— SERVES 4-6 ——

3 tbsp ghee

1 brown onion, peeled and diced

3 garlic cloves, crushed

1kg (2.2lb) grass-fed lamb mince

2 medium carrots, peeled and diced

2 cups (500ml) beef stock

½ cup (125ml) red wine

4 tbsp tomato paste

1 cinnamon quill

½ tsp allspice

1 tsp salt

2 bay leaves

2 tsp arrowroot powder

2 large sweet potatoes, peeled and chopped into small chunks

1. Heat 1 tbsp ghee over medium-high and sauté the onion and garlic until soft and translucent.

2. Add the lamb mince and stir frequently until lightly browned on all sides (about 10 minutes).

3. Add the carrot, stock, wine, tomato paste, spices, salt and bay leaves. Mix well and reduce to a low simmer. Cover and cook for 35 minutes, stirring occasionally.

4. After 35 minutes, add 1tbsp ghee and the arrowroot powder. Mix through for a minute until slightly thickened. Cook for a further few minutes uncovered and turn the heat off.

5. Place sweet potato in a saucepan and cover with water. Bring to the boil and cook for 15-20 minutes until soft.

6. Drain well and mash with 1 tbsp ghee and salt to taste.

7. Heat the oven to 200°C/390°F.

8. Spoon the lamb mixture into the bottom of small ovenproof ramekins, filling them about ¾ full. Spread the mash on top of the lamb to fill the dishes and scrape with a fork to rough up the top surface.

9. Bake for 10-15 minutes, and then place under a hot grill for 5 minutes to toast the top of the potato.

If you don't have small ramekins, use a large baking dish instead.

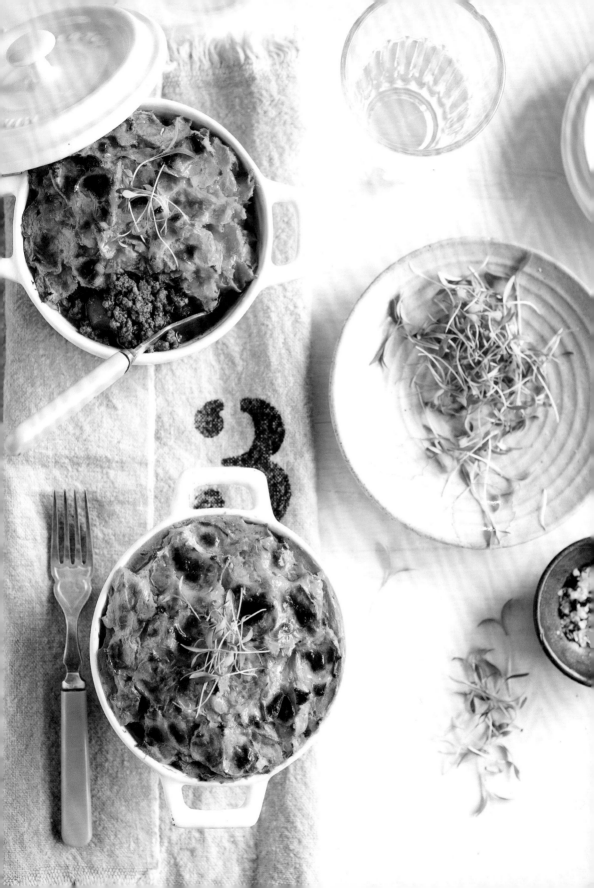

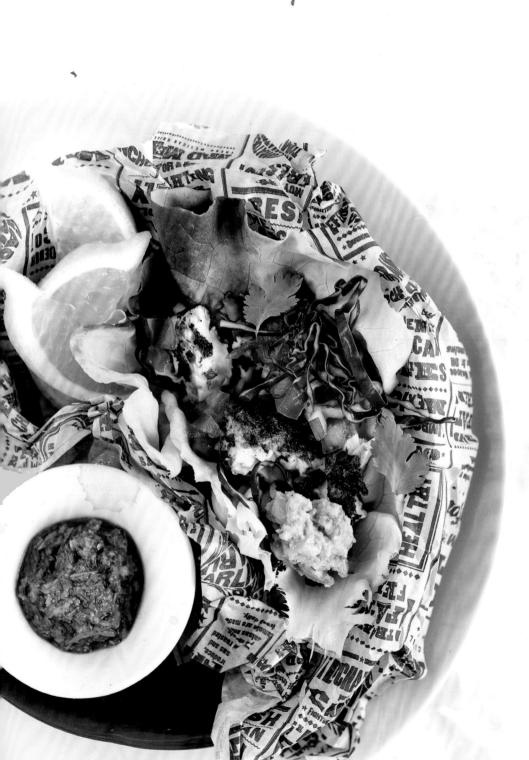

Chermoula fish tacos

700g (1.5lb) white fish fillets (halibut or similar)

1 Spanish (red) onion, peeled and diced

3 vine ripened tomatoes, diced

1 serving guacamole (page 58)

1 head of iceberg or butter lettuce

¼ head of red cabbage, finely sliced

2 tbsp coconut oil

CHERMOULA

¼ cup (5g) chopped fresh coriander

¼ cup (5g) chopped fresh parsley

⅓ cup (79ml) macadamia nut oil

2 garlic cloves, chopped

1 whole small red chilli, chopped

Zest of two lemons

¼ cup (60ml) lemon juice

1 tbsp ground cumin

2 tsp ground coriander

2 tsp smoked paprika

1 tsp salt

1. To make the seasoning, add all Chermoula ingredients into a food processor or similar and pulse until a thick paste forms.

2. Add salt and pepper to taste.

3. Lay all fish fillets flat in a non-metallic dish. Baste with half of the Chermoula mixture. Flip each fillet and baste the remaining puree over the fish so that all sides are seasoned. Marinate for at least a couple of hours in the refrigerator.

4. Meanwhile, arrange all the taco fillers on a large serving platter.

5. Wash and separate the iceberg or butter lettuce into large leaves to act as tortillas.

6. Heat a large pan on medium heat. Add the coconut oil and fry the fillets in batches until just cooked through (around 5 minutes).

7. Place the cooked fish in a serving dish and use a knife or spatula to gently flake into smaller pieces.

8. Place all ingredients in the middle of the table for a DIY taco feast!

Sticky apple pork ribs

—— SERVES 4 ——

Apple and pork are a delicious combination, and nothing beats a platter of sticky ribs to share with your friends or family. This recipe has the best of both worlds; a sticky apple-based sauce and tender meat that will easily pull away from the bone. Any extra sauce will keep in the refrigerator for up to 4 days.

1 cup (240g) unsweetened apple sauce

¼ cup coconut aminos

4 tbsp tomato puree

2 tbsp raw honey

2 tbsp apple cider vinegar

1 tbsp Dijon-style mustard

1 tsp dried oregano leaves

1 tsp smoked paprika

1 tsp ground ginger

½ tsp ground cumin

2 pork rib racks

500ml (2 cups) water

1. Preheat the oven to 220°C/425°F with a rack in the centre.

2. In a small saucepan over low heat, combine the apple sauce, coconut aminos, tomato puree, honey, apple cider vinegar, mustard, oregano and spices.

3. Bring to the boil then reduce to a low simmer for 5-10 minutes, or until the sauce starts to thicken.

4. Place the ribs on a rack in a roasting dish with the water in the bottom. Brush a small amount of the sauce onto both sides of the ribs but reserve most of it.

5. Cover the ribs in aluminium foil and roast for about 1½ hours, until the meat is tender and separates easily.

6. Remove the foil and transfer the ribs onto a flat tray lined with baking paper. Baste with remaining sticky sauce on both sides.

7. Cook uncovered for about 10 minutes or until the sauce is brown and sizzling.

8. Allow the ribs to rest for 10 minutes before slicing.

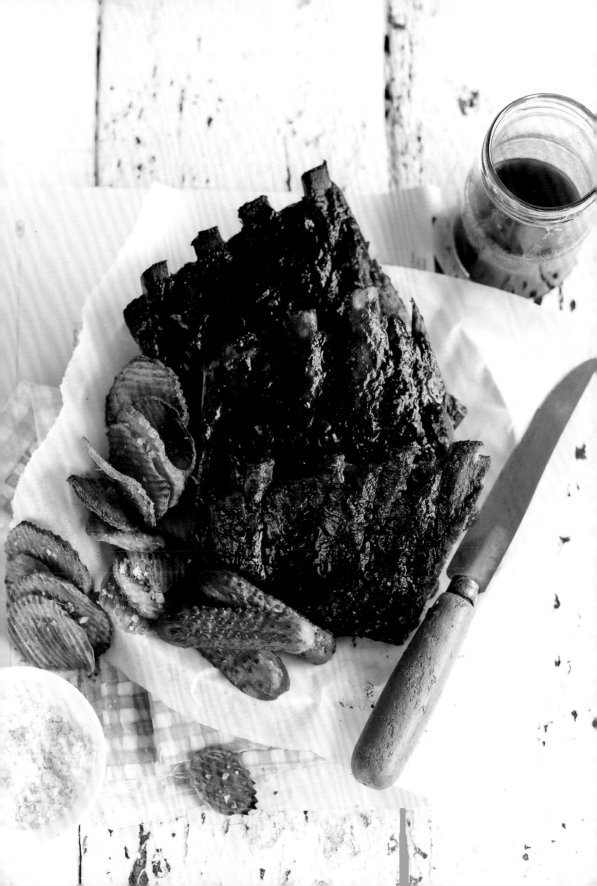

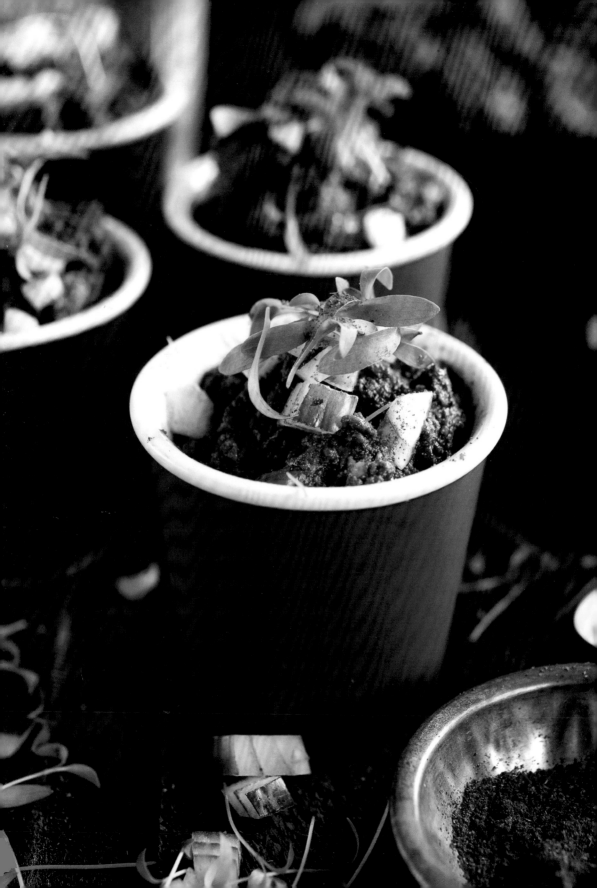

Chunky chilli con carne

1kg (2lb) grass-fed beef steak, diced (chuck or stew meat)

500g (1lb) grass-fed beef mince

1 tbsp dried oregano

1½ tbsp ground cumin

2-3 tbsp macadamia nut oil

2 white onions, diced

4 garlic cloves, crushed

800g (1.8lb) canned diced plum tomatoes

3 tbsp tomato paste

4-5 tbsp chilli sauce (find one with no sugar or preservatives)

½ tsp cayenne pepper

1 tbsp raw cacao powder

Salt to taste

Fresh cilantro (coriander) and diced Spanish (red) onion to serve

1. In a large mixing bowl coat the diced beef and mince with oregano and ground cumin.

2. In a large cast iron pot, heat the oil over medium-high heat. Add meat and stir for 2 minutes until brown almost all over.

3. Add the diced onions and garlic and stir for another 3 minutes or so until the onion is translucent and fragrant.

4. Add the canned tomatoes, tomato paste, chilli sauce, cayenne pepper and raw cacao. Adjust the amount of chilli to suit your preference.

5. Reduce to a simmer (there should be just enough liquid to cover the meat, but if it's looking dry, add some more tomato paste or a little water).

6. Simmer on low for 3-5 hours until the beef chunks start to break down.

This chilli is delicious on top of a baked sweet potato, folded in lettuce cups, on its own or as a healthy nachos topping! Serve with diced red onions and fresh coriander.

Ginger chilli chicken

This is a favourite marinade for chicken but also works well with beef and prawns. It's a great idea to make a big batch and store in the refrigerator for a fast, easy and delicious source of protein.

½ cup (125ml) tamari (wheat-free soy sauce)

1 tsp sesame oil

3cm (3 tbsp) fresh ginger, peeled and finely grated

2 garlic cloves, crushed

Rind of ½ lemon

Juice from ½ lemon

1 small fresh red chilli, finely chopped

2 tbsp sesame seeds

6 chicken drumsticks

1. Measure all marinade ingredients into a non-metallic, ovenproof dish and stir well.

2. Add the chicken drumsticks and flip a few times to coat them in marinade. Cover and set in the refrigerator for at least three hours.

3. Before cooking, bring the chicken to room temperature. Preheat the oven to 180°C/355°F.

4. Bake for 30-35 minutes, until browned and cooked through. Remove from the oven and let cool.

5. Serve with a big pile of roast veggies or on top of your favourite salad mix for lunch.

This recipe works really well with chicken thighs too. I like to make a full tray of thighs, allow them to cool and then chop the chicken roughly to create a pre-made protein for salads and fast meals.

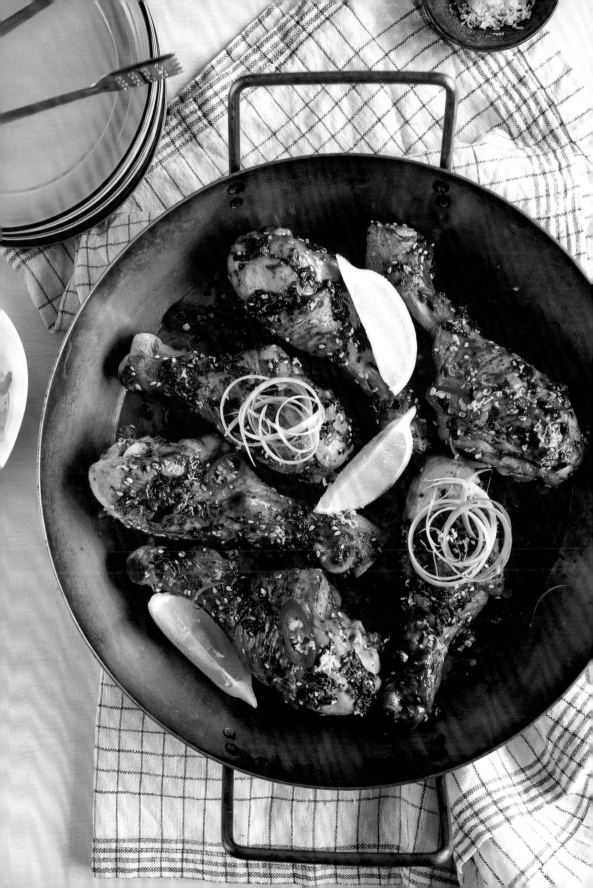

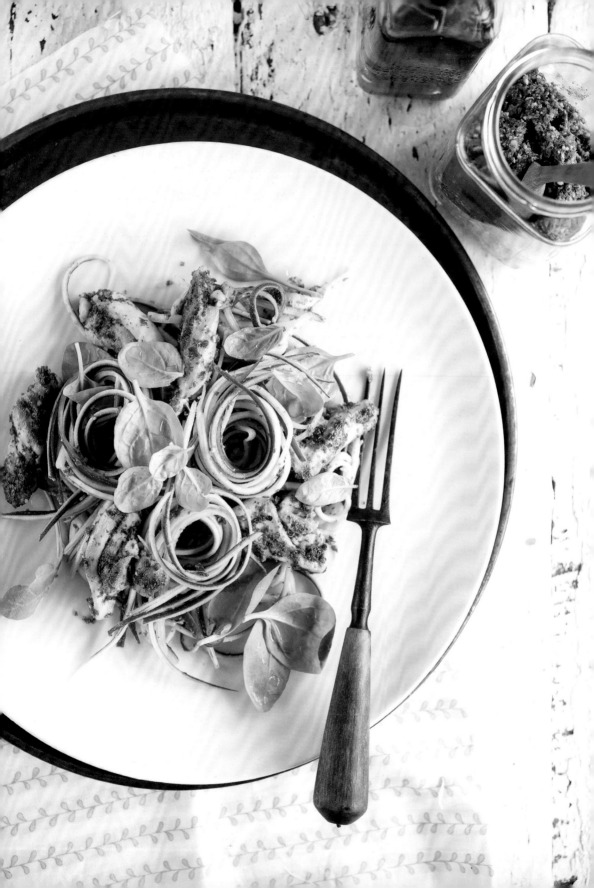

Chicken and kale pesto 'pasta'

—— **SERVES 2** ——

Zucchini 'noodles' are an amazing Paleo replacement for pasta, which is high on the list of inflammatory foods. This miraculous noodle substitute will inspire you to cut the pasta for good and get creative. This 'pasta' is delicious with meatballs, bolognaise and in salads too.

This is an easy and affordable meal that can be made in a matter of minutes, with some simple planning and meal preparation ahead of time. For a meat free lunch option, just two zucchini and some pre-made pesto is all you need!

4 green zucchinis
(courgettes)

1 tbsp coconut oil or ghee

2 skinless chicken thigh
fillets, quartered

¼ cup (65g) kale and basil
pesto

Handful of spinach leaves
to serve

KALE AND
BASIL PESTO

1 basil plant or large bunch,
large stems removed

¾ cup (177ml) extra virgin
olive oil

3 large kale (Tuscan
cabbage) leaves,
de-stemmed and chopped
(about 1.5 cups/100g)

½ cup (80g) raw cashews

¼ cup (30g) pistachios

1 tbsp chopped mint

Salt, to taste

1. Place all the pesto ingredients in a food processor and pulse until smooth. Scrape into an airtight jar and keep in the refrigerator.

2. Roughly peel the zucchini and chop off both ends. Using a handheld julienne device or vegetable spiraliser, process the zucchinis into noodle-like pasta, discard the core (or use it in your next green smoothie!).

3. Heat the oil in a pan on medium-high. Add the chicken, turning regularly until browned and cooked through, about 10 minutes.

4. Add the pre-made pesto and stir for 1 minute to coat the chicken.

5. Add the zucchini and stir for another minute. Turn off the heat and dish into bowls immediately to prevent the zucchini from turning soggy.

SWEETER TREATS

Barbecued pineapple skewers

Watermelon and basil granita

Banana and macadamia 'ice-cream'

Chewy mocha powerballs

Lemon thyme roast peaches with vanilla cashew cream

The primal mess

Strawberry and green tea icy poles

You will notice that there aren't a large amount of Paleo desserts in this section. Although sweeter treats are a part of life and popular in Paleo cooking sources, I wanted this book to represent a balanced and sugar-free approach to everyday life. Many people who experience a transition into a primal way of living will kick their sugar habit, and therefore not crave as many sweets and treats throughout the day. If we start to introduce Paleo desserts that use a large amount of 'natural' sugars, we can continue to fuel our reward response and fuel an addiction to sugar without realising it. The desserts in this section are mostly based on whole-fruit and crowd-pleasers that you can bring to your next barbecue or make for an after-school treat for your kids. As they contain no hidden, refined or artificial sugars, these sweeter treats are suitable for the occasional morning teas, boosts of energy and fuel for exercise. It might be helpful to have some of these options around the house when you first transition into the Paleo diet, as you may find it harder to kick the sugar habit than you think!

Barbecued pineapple skewers

—— SERVES 4 ——

2 medium pineapples, peeled with tops removed

8 skewers (metal preferred)

¼ cup (85g) raw honey

Juice from 1 lime (3 tbsp)

Handful fresh mint leaves, to garnish

1. Remove the middle core of each pineapple and chop the flesh into bite-sized cubes.

2. Thread the pineapple pieces onto the skewers and place in a shallow baking dish.

3. In a small pitcher, mix the honey and lime juice and pour evenly over the skewers. Leave to marinate in the refrigerator for a couple of hours.

4. On a medium heat, barbecue the skewers for 3-5 minutes with the lid closed. When ready, they should be slightly caramelised and soft.

5. Allow to cool then garnish with fresh mint and slices of lime.

Other sweet fruits are delicious caramelised on the BBQ too! Try juicy peaches or apricots.

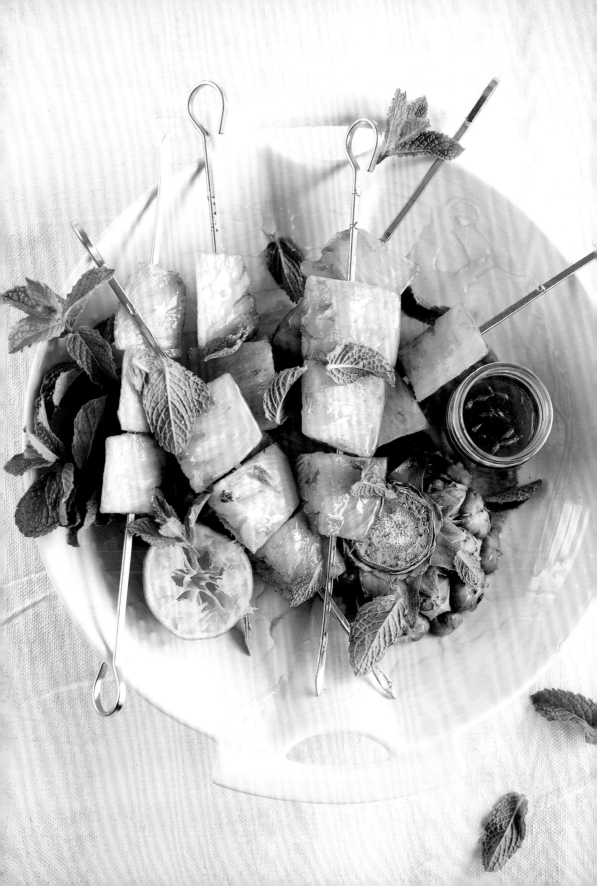

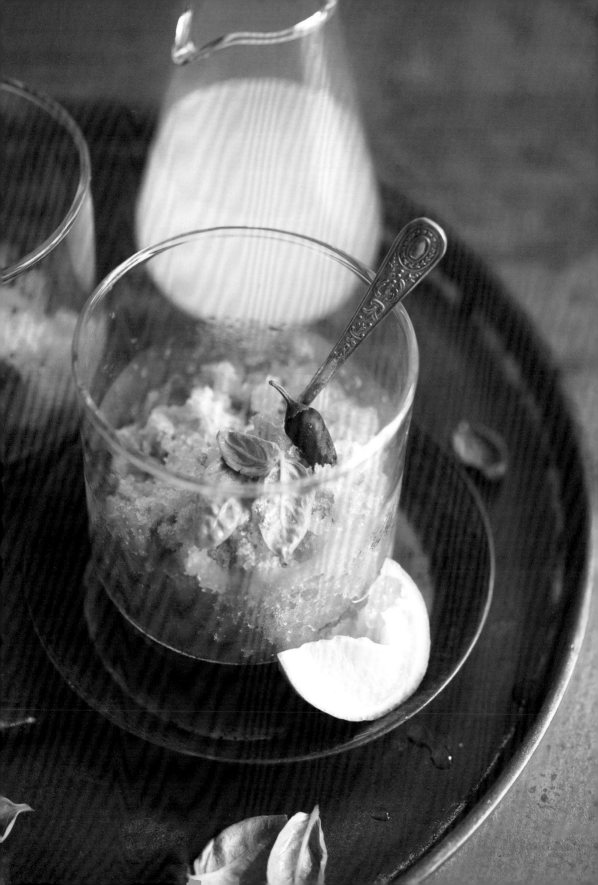

Watermelon and basil granita

2 cups frozen, cubed watermelon

½ small red chilli or ½ tsp chilli flakes (optional)

5 basil leaves, plus a few for serving

Lime rind and salt, to serve (optional)

1. In a food processor, pulse all ingredients to slowly break up the frozen watermelon. Over-process and you will end up with fancy watermelon juice!

2. Just as it reaches a sorbet-like consistency, scoop into small bowls and top with some basil sprigs.

At your next trip to the Farmer's market, stock up on cheap, in-season fruit like watermelon or peaches. Peel, dice and freeze in sealed bags or containers for a quick and easy dessert like this.

Banana and macadamia 'ice-cream'

3 frozen bananas, chopped

2 tbsp macadamia nut butter (or another nut butter if you prefer)

¼ cup (60ml) coconut cream (chilled)

Desiccated coconut to serve

A few raw macadamias, chopped

1. Place all the ingredients, except the chopped nuts, into the large bowl of a food processor. Pulse until just blended to reach the consistency of ice cream. Avoid over blending and melting the mixture.

2. Top with the chopped nuts and a little cinnamon if you like!

You can store leftovers (if there are any!) in the freezer for a quick dessert later. The mixture can freeze quite solid, so leave it to soften a little before digging in.

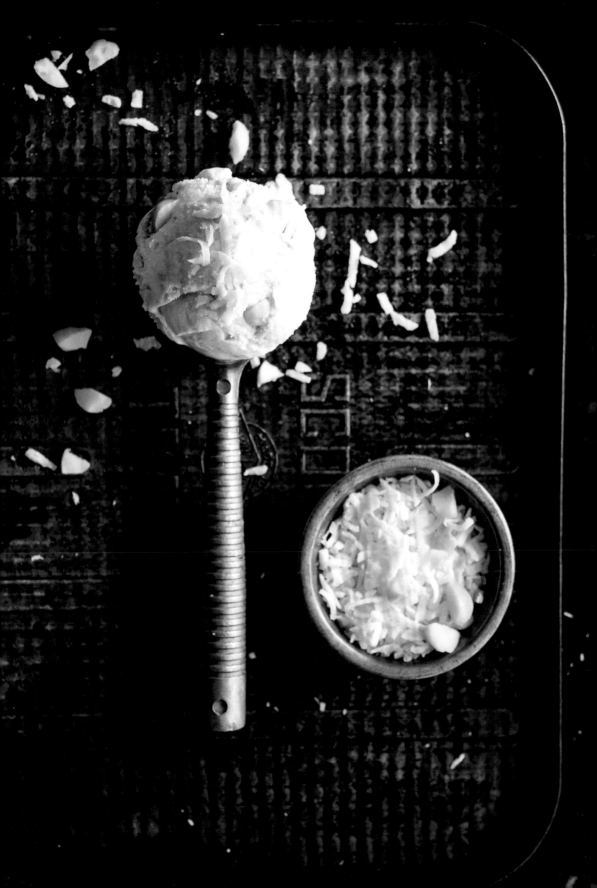

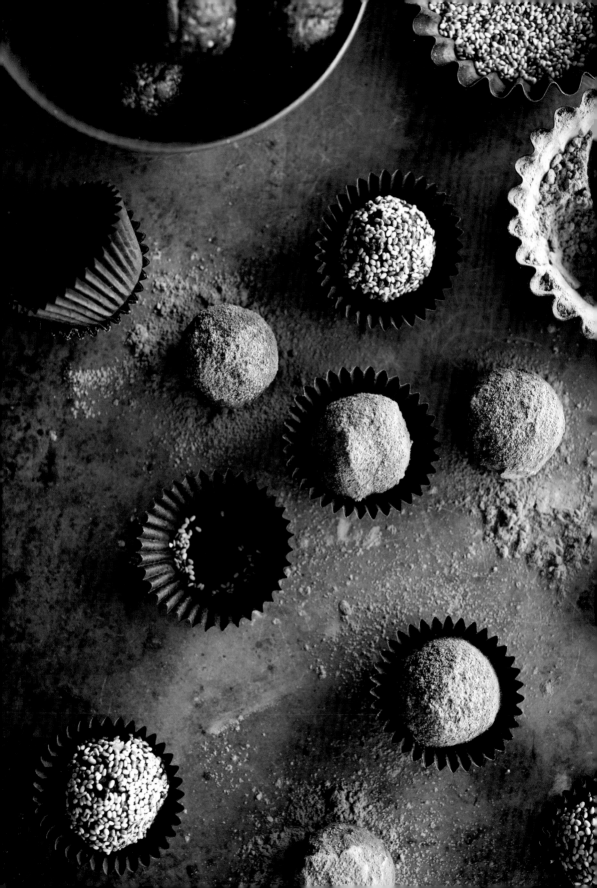

Chewy mocha powerballs

1 cup raw nuts (e.g. a mix of macadamia and cashew, almonds, walnuts or pecans)

8 fresh Medjool dates, pitted

2 tbsp raw cacao powder

3cm (3tbsp) chunk ginger, finely grated

2 tbsp coconut oil, melted

1 tbsp coconut flakes

1 tbsp cinnamon

1 tsp salt

1 tbsp finely ground coffee beans

2 heaping tbsp goji berries

PLUS, FOR DUSTING:

¼ cup (37g) chia seeds

¼ cup (30g) raw cacao powder

1. In a food processor, add the nuts and pulse until roughly ground but still chunky.

2. Add the pitted dates, cacao powder, ginger, coconut oil, coconut flakes, cinnamon, salt, and coffee. Process until the mixture is starting to stick together (about 60 seconds on high).

3. Add the goji berries and pulse for 15 seconds.

4. Pour the dusting chia seeds and cacao onto two plates.

5. Using your hands, roll the mixture into small balls (about 3cm/ 1 inch across).

6. Roll the balls in the toppings to coat the outer surface.

7. Place in a single layer on a flat plate and set in the refrigerator or freezer until eaten.

The coffee in this recipe is added mainly to create a coffee-chocolate flavour, which is intensified when chilled. If serving in the afternoon or evening, omit the coffee to prevent sleepless nights!

Lemon thyme roast peaches with vanilla cashew cream

4 peaches

1 tbsp maple syrup

Small bunch of fresh lemon thyme, plus extra to serve

6 tbsp cashew cream (page 46)

1. Preheat the oven to 220°C/425°F and line a flat tray with baking paper.

2. Slice each peach in half and remove the stones. Place on baking tray cut-side up, drizzle with maple syrup and sprinkle with lemon thyme.

3. Roast for 20 minutes or until peaches are soft and starting to caramelise. They should still hold their shape.

4. When making the cashew cream add 1 Medjool date and vanilla from one fresh pod into the blender with the cashews.

5. For each serving, top two peach halves with a dollop of cashew cream and a sprinkle of fresh thyme.

You could easily substitute the cashew cream in this recipe for chilled coconut cream.

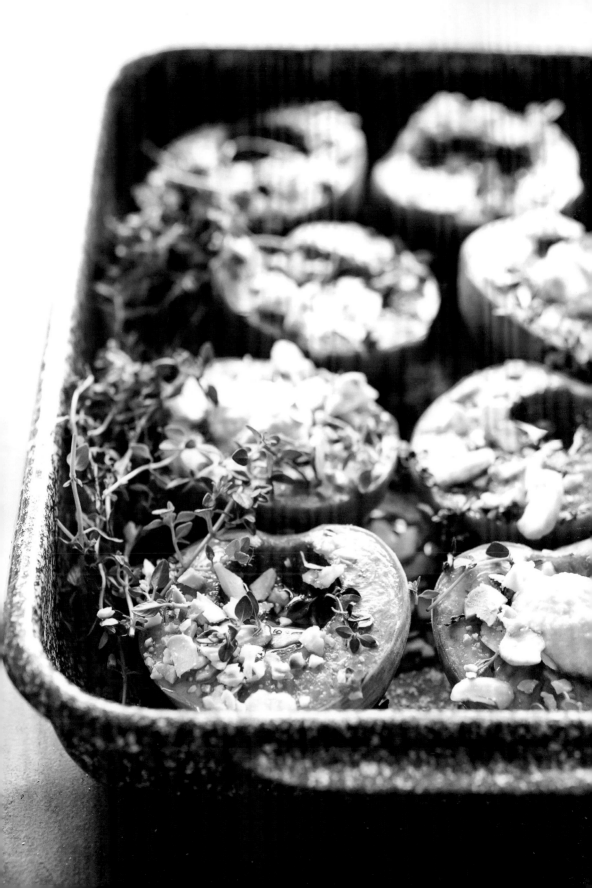

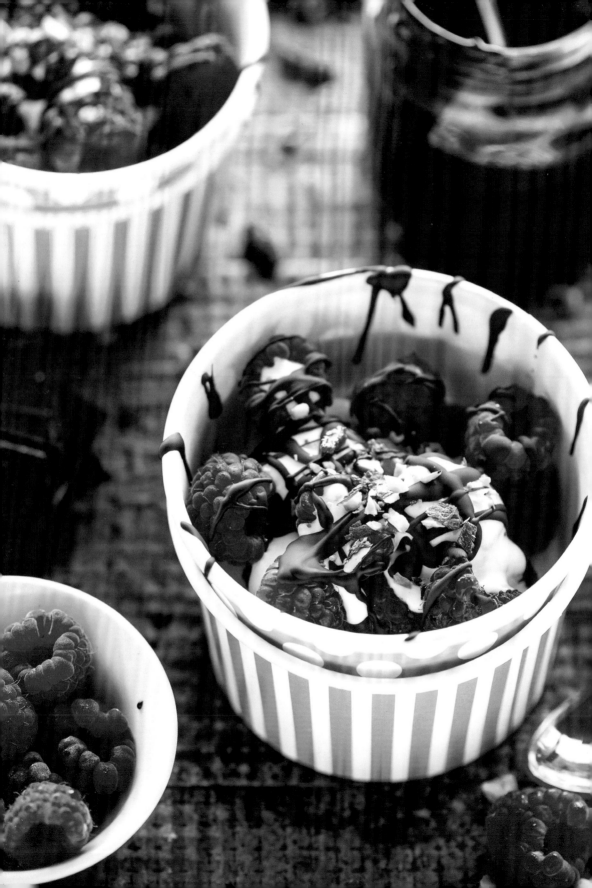

The primal mess

This is a favourite fast and messy dessert that hits the spot when you're looking for an after dinner treat. It was modelled on a dessert called The Eton Mess, a mish-mash of meringue, cream and a post consumption sugar crash!

50g dark chocolate, minimum 85% cacao

1 cup (130g) frozen raspberries

2 tbsp coconut cream (or cashew cream from page 46)

Sea salt

1 tbsp goji berries

2 tbsp chopped pistachios

1. Melt the chocolate in a double boiler or on low power in the microwave. Be careful not to burn it.

2. Divide the frozen raspberries into two bowls and add 1 tbsp coconut or cashew cream into each.

3. Spoon the melted chocolate evenly on top of the raspberries and immediately sprinkle the goji berries, pistachios and sea salt into each bowl.

4. As the chocolate cools, it will harden and form a shell that you can crack with a spoon!

Get creative with your Primal mess! Delicious additions include coconut flakes, chopped nuts, herbs and a variety of frozen fruits as a base.

Strawberry and green tea icy poles

2 tea bags of high quality green tea

4 cups (1 litre) filtered water (boiled to 80°C/176°F to prevent making the tea bitter)

2 cups (250g) frozen strawberries, plus about 6 berries kept in chunks/halves

1. In a large jug or glass jar, simmer the green tea in the water until it reaches desired strength (around 5 minutes). Remove the tea bags and allow to cool.

2. In a blender or food processor, puree the strawberries with about 2 tbsp of water.

3. Divide the pureed strawberries into the bottom of the Popsicle moulds.

4. Carefully pour in the green tea to top off each mould and drop a whole berry into each one before inserting the handle.

5. Place in the freezer overnight or until frozen solid.

6. Run warm water over the moulds before loosening and removing each popsicle.

Change up the flavours of your pops with different fruit purees and a variety of tea.

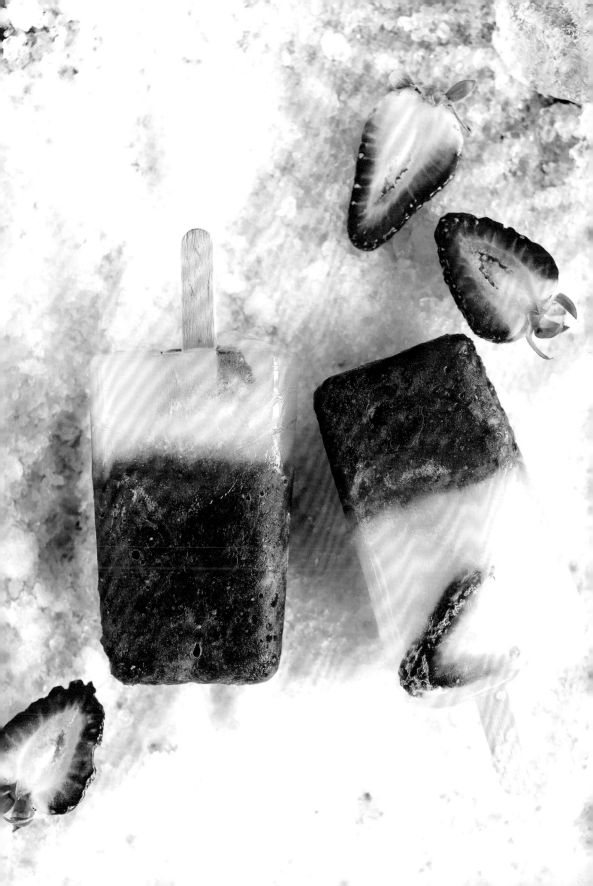

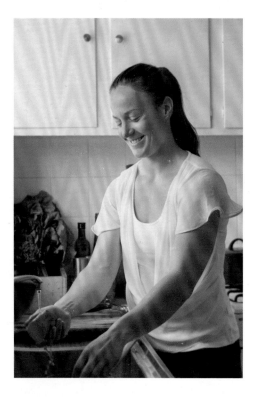

About The Author:

Elizabeth Marsh is a qualified sports scientist and personal trainer from New Zealand. She is currently based in Melbourne, Australia and has worked in the fitness industry for the past 7 years with both recreational and elite level athletes. Through the development of an online and educational community, Primal Junction, her goal is to challenge accepted nutritional and exercise guidelines and encourage individuals to take control of their life through a holistic understanding of real-food, natural human movement, hormonal health, stress reduction and community.

Website: *www.primaljunction.com*

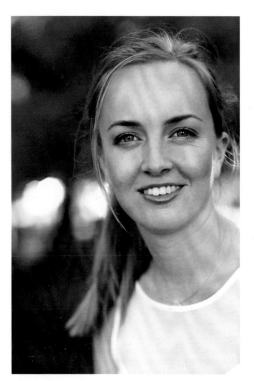

About The Photographer:

Rachel Jane is a self-taught food photographer and stylist based in Melbourne, Australia. As the creator of her beloved blog, Two Loves Studio, she shares her evolving journey into the world of food photography. She is passionate about shooting food portraiture that highlights the simplicity and beauty of real food. Her styling focuses on the shapes and textures of the recipe components, which allows us to connect with the dish and evokes our love affair with food.

Blog: *http://twolovesstudio.com*
Portfolio: *http://racheljane.photography*
Instagram: *http://instagram.com/rjcam*